Time For Bed

Healthy Sleep Training from Birth to Five

BY

Mary Simmons

Copyright © 2019 by Mary Simmons

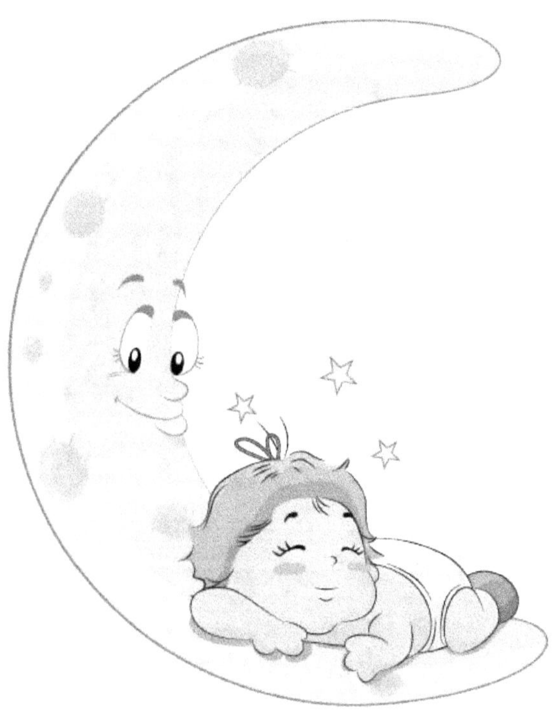

Disclaimer

All the material contained in this book is provided for educational and informational purposes only. No responsibility can be taken for any results or outcomes resulting from the use of this material. While every attempt has been made to provide information that is both accurate and effective, the author does not assume any responsibility for the misuse of this information.

BONUS

Here's your bonus
http://marysimmonsbook.com/home/

Table of Contents

PREFACE

This book serves as a manual on how to sleep train your child successfully with carefully researched tips and instructions which have professional backing. The proper steps to take in sleep training and the common challenges are examined with in-depth solutions given.

Common myths and wrong assertions concerning sleep training are also examined and debunked. The steps and methods are easy to understand and are also child friendly. This book is useful for parents and intended parents alike.

INTRODUCTION

Sleep is one of the most important ways to ensure healthy living. It is also very important for your child's growth and development. This is particularly seen in newborns, who, as you'll notice, generally sleep for most of the day. Sleep is directly involved in brain development in children and to an extent in adults. During sleep, the body takes its time to "get rid of the trash." It is when the body repairs itself and flushes toxins away. The body also produces hormones that are necessary for growth and development during sleep.

Since babies are still growing, they might need some help getting to sleep and sleeping for the right amount of time. A good sleep will directly influence your child's mood and behavior, as is also the case with adults. You are more likely to feel alert and well rested after getting a good night's sleep or a good nap than when you stay up all night. Researchers have also discovered that sleep directly affects growth. Children who are consistently sleep deprived have an increased chance of suffering from growth hormone deficiency. This is why newborns spend half of their day sleeping.

Babies between 0-5 years might experience trouble with sleeping or maintaining a bedtime routine. This can affect not only the baby negatively, but also you as the parent. Most times, babies who have trouble falling asleep at night will do the next thing common to them—cry. This can get frustrating for a lot of parents as both you and a crying baby won't experience a good night's rest. Imagine trying to pacify a crying baby after a stressful day at work. It doesn't sound nice, does it?

This is why sleep training is very important. Up to 30 percent of children will have problems with falling asleep or staying asleep. They will then need additional help from the parents to make sure they get the right amount of sleep each day. It is important to check whether your child gets enough sleep each day. You as the parent must help them maintain proper sleeping habits. Your child shouldn't have access to electronic devices at night, and the other members of the household need to cooperate to help maintain a peaceful environment that will help the baby sleep better.

Babies between 0-2 months should get around 10 to 18 hours of sleep per day, according to the National Sleep Foundation. From 3 to 12 months, 9.5 to 14 hours is enough. Children 1-3 years old should get between 12 to 14 hours of sleep each day, while 11-13 hours is adequate for 3- to 5-year-olds.

It is important to choose the right sleep training approach for your baby, as choosing the wrong methods may have the opposite effect. In this book, we'll examine the best methods to help your child get the amount of sleep that is recommended by pediatricians.

PART ONE

***

WHAT TO KNOW BEFORE YOU START

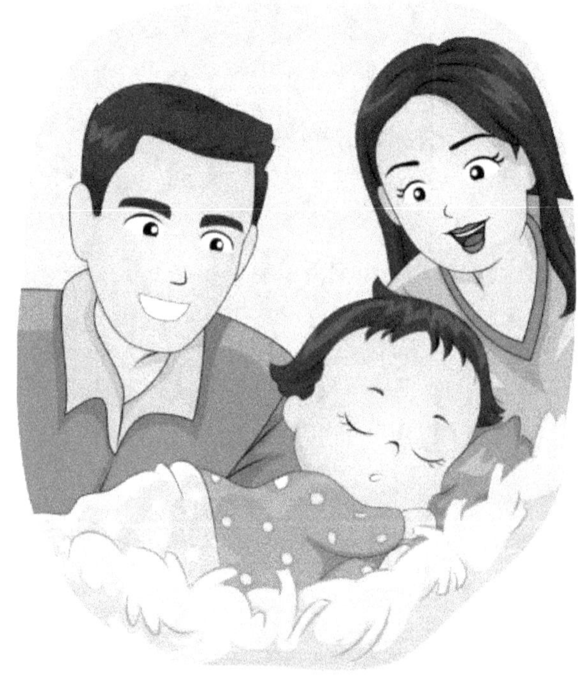

efore you start sleep training for your baby, there are some important things you should know. First, it is important to make sure **your child is ready for sleep**

training. Most experts agree that babies are usually ready between **four to six months old**. Around this time, babies start to develop a **circadian rhythm** (an internal body clock that regulates a 24-hour cycle of biological processes). They start to have usual sleep and wake times. This might not be always constant, but it should be noticeable by now. Your baby should also be able to sleep for long hours continuously each night. You should also note that babies are not the same, so you should **adjust your methods and timing** to suit your baby's needs.

*A child is ready for sleep
training around 4-6 mo*

You must be prepared as a parent to help your baby maintain a consistent and uninterrupted bedtime routine. Sleep training isn't just about encouraging your baby to sleep at a particular time; it also involves creating a conducive environment for the baby to sleep without interruption. There are many methods commonly used in sleep training for babies but you should try one which is **convenient for both** you and the baby.

Another thing you should know is that sleep training is different for each baby. Some do not require a lot of time before they start sleeping at the right periods, while it might take weeks for others to adapt. You must also be prepared for regressions, as some factors might affect the child's sleep later on. For example, a child might find it difficult to fall asleep when in a new environment and also if there is a break in bedtime routines. Illness may also affect a baby's sleep routine. It is also common for babies to have trouble sleeping during the teething process.

It might be beneficial to combine different methods of getting a baby to maintain a proper sleep process, provided that the methods are recommended by pediatricians and are not inconvenient for the baby. It may look like you are not getting results at first, which is why **consistency is key**. You should try to understand your baby and adopt a sleep training method that is best for him. Do not start sleep training when both you and the child are not ready. The process might not be successful at the end or it might take longer than usual if this happens.

Consistency is Key

When the baby is ready for sleep training, there are some items you need to get and some bedtime routines you can follow to make the process easier and faster. For example, a baby monitor is an important item to have when you start sleep training. If you will be using the no-tears method, then you must be prepared to spend a lot of time with your baby each night. It may also take a longer time than most other methods of sleep training, though it will be worth it in the long run. You can also check if there are any health issues that may cause sleeping problems.

What is Healthy Sleep?

Before you can say your child has had a good night's sleep, there are some factors you must consider. These are the essentials of healthy sleep. We'll go through them one by one so you will know what to look out for to be sure your child acquires a healthy sleep pattern. The first thing that establishes a healthy sleep pattern is getting the recommended amount of sleep each day.

> *According to the National Sleep Foundation,*
>
> *children should get*
>
> *10-18 hours when 0-2 months old;*
>
> *9.5-14 hours when 3-12 months old;*
>
> *12-14 hours when 1-3 years old;*
>
> *11-13 hours when 3-5 years old.*

A healthy sleep also follows the normal circadian rhythm, which involves sleeping at the right period for the right amount of time. A child who sleeps well during the day but has trouble sleeping at night can't be said to have a healthy sleep pattern, even though he makes up the time by napping. A child should be able to fall asleep at the period appropriate for their age group.

Healthy sleep also involves sleeping without many breaks or interruptions. Your baby should be able to sleep for long stretches each night without crying or waking up and later experiencing difficulty falling asleep. Healthy sleep also means the absence of snoring, difficulty breathing, and other sleeping problems. When your baby is able to sleep through the night without exhibiting restlessness and experiencing sleep disturbances, he can then be said to have healthy sleep. Snoring and breathing difficulties are common sleeping problems seen in both children and adults. Often, these problems may be an indication of other underlying health problems such as sleep apnea.

Healthy sleep also involves **sleeping through the night** or during the day without external disturbances. Noise, bright lights, heat, and cold all can affect a baby's sleep. To sleep properly, a baby should be in an environment that's free from noise and isn't too hot or too cold. These external factors can cause a baby to wake up at different times and will not allow for a healthy sleep.

A healthy sleep is sleep through the night

Another way to check for healthy sleep is to look out for how the **baby behaves** when he **wakes up**. A healthy sleep should leave the baby **feeling refreshed**, calm and alert. A baby who wakes up feeling groggy, irritable or screaming can't be said to have had a good sleep.

Healthy sleep also involves going through the normal four sleep stages. The first stage is light sleep. It is common to experience shakes and jerks which might easily disrupt the sleep process. The second stage involves a steady decrease in body temperature, heartrate, and brain activity. The third stage involves little brain activity and it is difficult to wake from. The last stage is REM sleep, which stands for Rapid Eye Movement. This is when dreams start to occur and eye movements get rapid. Though it is easy to awaken at this stage, the person still feels sleepy or groggy.

Benefits of Healthy Sleep

The benefits of healthy sleep cannot be overstated, since sleep is an integral part of a baby's growth and development. Children who get the right amount of sleep have better mental and physical health. A sleep-deprived child will experience attention and behavioral problems. A child who sleeps for the recommended amount of hours will be more alert and cheerful than a child who has stayed awake through the night. Such a child will be irritable and difficult to pacify. A sleep-deprived child will also experience learning difficulties which might progress into anxiety and depression later on.

Sleep is essential for a baby's growth and development

A healthy sleep allows for the body to repair damaged tissue and ensure **muscle growth**. Essential growth hormones are also released during sleep. It has been discovered that children who experience problems sleeping over a long period of time might suffer from growth hormone deficiency, as the body does not have the opportunity to release enough growth hormones. A healthy sleep also helps in developing a **strong immune system**. Children who are sleep deprived may be more susceptible to illnesses such as the flu and the common cold. Good sleep also helps in maintaining a **healthy body weight**, as children who get less than the recommended amount of sleep each day have a higher chance of being obese.

Proper sleep also helps to **reduce stress levels** in both children and adults. Sleep deprivation leads to irritability and tiredness, which in turn to leads to frustration. During sleep, the brain regulates memories and strengthens the bond between neurons. This is why it is easier to learn something new just after waking up from a good sleep. Healthy sleep will help to consolidate skills learned while awake. A healthy sleep helps you feel refreshed and mentally alert. Sleep-deprived children will often experience learning difficulties.

Your child's quality of life can be affected either positively or negatively by sleep. Studies have been made which show the relationship between healthy sleep and a long lifespan, although it hasn't been determined if it is the cause or an effect.

Healthy sleep also helps to **prevent heart disease, stroke, diabetes, and arthritis**. Lack of sleep is linked to an increase in inflammatory proteins, which contribute to various health issues. Sleep deprivation also causes an increase in the C-reactive protein, which can increase the risk of getting a heart attack.

A healthy sleep also influences the overall health of your family. A sleep-deprived baby who cries through the night will be a source of worry to the whole family and will likely cause other members of the family to also suffer from sleep deprivation. Sleep training is necessary for your infant to get enough sleep, your whole family to remain healthy and happy, and for you to have stress-free days.

Research on Children's Sleep

A lot of research has been done on children's sleep by reputable child care specialists which will go a long way in helping you choose the right sleep training method for your child.

Michelle Drerup, Psy.D, the director of Behavioral Sleep Medicine at Cleveland Clinic, says that getting less than six hours of sleep per night is connected to having a lower immunity response and increased risk of cardiovascular incidents. It also leads to a higher metabolism rate and can affect the production of hormones negatively. Likewise, Dr. Suresh Kotagal, a child neurologist and also a pediatric sleep specialist at the Mayo Clinic, opines that sleep deprivation can affect the frontal lobes in children, which then impacts mood, attention, and concentration. Sleep deprivation often leads to a wrong diagnosis of Attention Deficit Disorder. Sometimes the child is just sleep deprived. Even children who really have ADD or ADHD often experience a sleep disorder.

Sleep expert and university professor Wendy Hall conducted a study to check out how technology use affects children's sleep. It was discovered that the more exposed a child is to electronic gadgets close to bedtime, the less amount of sleep they get. Maintaining good sleep hygiene practices is very important in making sure children get a good night's sleep.

According to Marc Weissbluth, MD, good sleep helps to increase brainpower just like weight lifting increases muscle power. It can **increase a child's attention span** and help the child relax physically, as well as improving the child's mental alertness. He defines sleep as a power source that helps to keep the mind alert and calm. In his study, he also made some other observations concerning children's sleep. First, sleep problems in children cannot be outgrown; they need to be dealt with.

Weissbluth stated that children who sleep during the day will have longer attention spans than children who do not. Children who have a healthy sleep routine are less demanding and do not throw tantrums as much as children who are sleep-deprived. Long-term sleep deprivation also shows serious effects on brain function. In each age group, it was discovered that children who are more intelligent slept longer than those who weren't. Good sleep also improved classroom performance and social relations in children with attention deficit hyperactivity disorder. Many behavioral problems and learning difficulties can be avoided through healthy sleep. Healthy sleep affects neurological development positively.

The Importance of Family Harmony and Support

Family support and harmony are very important in sleep training. It is not just the responsibility of you as the parent. Other members of the household must be prepared to modify their sleep schedules in order to help you and the baby go through the sleep training process.

One of the major roles of other family members during a child's sleep training is to help maintain a perfect environment for the child to have a good sleep when it's bedtime or nap time. It is advisable to choose a sleep training method that will work for both the baby and the rest of the household, and for every member to agree upon the sleep training method to be used. It is not a good idea for each person to try their own method. This doesn't mean that every member of the family should not be involved with the process; rather, it means cooperation is very important for sleep training to be successful.

A family with a sleep trained baby will be at rest. It can be a frustrating and tiring process, and when the baby cries during the night, undoubtedly the stress levels of everyone in the family will increase. This is why everyone should work together to make sure the baby gets sleep trained successfully as quickly as possible.

For families with working parents, each member of the household must be aware of the sleep training routine and must be prepared to help in the absence of a parent. The family member in charge of the baby should also stick strictly to the previous sleep training routine adopted for the baby. Just as the members of the family work together to ensure the baby's safety, they should also work together to make sure the baby gets good sleep each day. The burden of sleep training shouldn't be on only one member of the family; all members should work together.

When it's bedtime, family members should be ready to make the environment conducive for the baby. No loud noises or music. The lights should be dimmed to help the baby sleep properly. If the baby stays in its own room, other family members should only go in once the baby is sleeping and be as silent as possible.

During sleep training for toddlers, other members of the family shouldn't encourage bad sleep habits. A child will go to sleep faster when it's bedtime if the whole family goes to sleep or maintains a silent atmosphere. Your toddler will find it hard to sleep if there's another family member playing loud music in the next room or talking loudly. **Family harmony and support really goes a long way in ensuring the success of sleep training.**

How Parents Can Prepare Themselves

Before starting sleep training, it is important to educate yourself and get yourself familiar with the process rather than just jumping into it. When you notice your child has trouble sleeping through the night or during the day, you should first check to see if there is an underlying medical condition that can cause sleep disorders. After making sure this is not the case, discuss sleep training methods with your pediatrician and other family members. You can then adopt a method that suits your baby. Another thing to note is that it is very important to make your sure your child is actually ready for sleep training before starting. Most children are ready somewhere between four to six months old.

You should also take note of how many hours of sleep your child gets each day. This enables you to prepare a suitable sleep training plan. If your child is getting the recommended amount of sleep without issues, then sleep training might not be necessary. Babies between 4 to 12 months old should get around 12-16 hours per day, according to the American Academy of Sleep Medicine.

To prepare yourself for sleep training, you can keep a **sleep log** to help you track your baby's sleeping pattern. This helps you determine when the baby usually goes to sleep and how many hours of sleep he gets each night. To prepare the baby, you should set a stable bedtime. Most people agree on between **seven or eight o'clock.** Together with this, you should also develop a bedtime routine, including activities that can soothe the baby and make him feel more relaxed, like massages, warm baths, and cradling.

> *Keep a sleep log to track your baby's sleeping pattern*

To further prepare for sleep training, you should speak with other members of the household or the caregiver to agree on the sleep training method and routines. They must be prepared to try their best in maintaining a conducive environment for the baby. You can also make yourself familiar with sleep training tools and gadgets. It is important to learn the safety rules and procedures for sleep training babies. For example, babies should not sleep face down in a crib; they should always sleep on their back. There should also be no objects left in the crib.

You should start sleep training at a time when it is convenient for you and the baby. If you can't be fully involved, get another family member to help you out. You might lose some sleep during the process so you must be prepared for that. Another important step is to prepare the sleep environment. If your child will be sleeping in a new place, it is best to prepare it and make the child familiar with it. After that, make sure the other items needed for sleep training are available.

*Start sleep training when it's
okay for you and the baby*

Sleep Training for Working Parents

If sleep training already looks difficult for stay-at-home parents, it might look impossible for working parents. Regardless, it is inevitable. If you are a working parent, you do not want to come back after a long day at work to cope with the stress of a crying baby at night. That is why sleep training is important either way. Sleep training for working parents actually isn't impossible, despite how hard it may seem. You may, however, have to employ some different methods and routines. You'll also need to share the training duties and responsibilities. It helps to create comfortable bedtime routines that suit the baby and at the same time is convenient for both of you. You may also need to enlist the help of other family members.

Structure the sleep training process in a way that doesn't affect your partner's sleep cycle. As we've said before, it is best to schedule the sleep training at a period when it's comfortable for you and the baby. Choose a starting time when you are less busy, such as during the weekend. Since most jobs offer maternity leave, you should take advantage of this period to start the sleep training process so by the time you return to work, your child is already sleep trained. Another factor to consider is consistency. **Do not start** the sleep training at a period **when you cannot be consistent with it**. It would amount to a waste of time if you do this. It is better to start when you can offer the utmost dedication to the sleep training routines or at a time when you have people or family members that can help you with it.

Before starting sleep training as a working parent, make sure you discuss the process, methods, and bedtime routines with your family members or the caregiver. This will make it easy for you as they can help ensure the methods are consistent in your absence. You should also make sure all the items needed for sleep training are available.

Each Child is Different

A common mistake parents make is to compare their child with other children. Some try to adopt the same sleep training method either a friend or relative used for their child, without considering their baby's personality and uniqueness. Even among siblings, you may need to adopt different methods and routines for each child. Each child has his own personality and it would be erroneous to use one approach for every child. Another thing you should know as a parent is that the sleep training period varies from child to child. While other children may go through the process within a few days or a week, other children might need as long as two weeks or more. There is no specific timeframe for sleep training. However, if the process seems to be taking longer than usual or if it shows no results after a long period of time, you might need to reevaluate your methods.

Research has also shown that the **baby's temperament can affect sleep training** and this should be considered by parents. Babies react to things in different ways. While one baby might cry loudly during the night because of a minor inconvenience, another baby might just wake up from sleep and stay quiet. The best thing is to study your child's temperament to help you determine the best sleep training method for him.

Once you know your child's temperament, it's easier to know what to do in certain situations. You'll be able to tell if the baby is hungry, cold, or uncomfortable rather than just guessing what's wrong.

Why Children Cry

This is one of the most common questions asked by frustrated parents. Sometimes it looks like your child just keeps crying for no reason, although this isn't true. Since babies are not yet developed enough to communicate verbally, crying is the only way available for them to communicate. It is up to the parents to find out why the baby is crying. It can be frustrating when your child wakes up everyone in the house with loud cries during the night and it doesn't seem like he is ever going to stop, but it is your job as the parent to figure out why and what to do to soothe him. We'll go through some major reasons children cry.

One of the main reasons children cry during sleep is if they are uncomfortable. Sometimes the baby has been in a single position for too long and it starts to get uncomfortable for him. Blood circulation may also be restricted to an area which will cause an uncomfortable sensation. What the parent needs to do is to simply move the baby a bit or lift him up gently. The baby might also turn around during sleep, in which case you could help him adjust to a more comfortable position.

Children also cry if they are injured, sick, or during teething. If your child cries too loudly for a long period of time or in an unusual manner, it is advisable to check his body for injuries, feel his temperature, or visit a doctor if necessary. Your baby will also cry if he is hungry, which is why you should always take a mental note of your child's feeding schedule. Once it's his usual feeding time, make sure you feed him.

Another reason children cry is if they are scared. Your child might wake up from sleep suddenly to a dark room or a strange environment, especially if he fell asleep in another location. All what you need to do is to soothe the child until he goes back to sleep. This and many other reasons may be the cause of your child's heartbreaking cries. You should study your child to enable you figure out the common reasons. You should visit a medical professional if there's anything unusual.

Things You Need For Successful Sleep Training

Before you begin sleep training, there are some supplies you should get. These include:

1. A baby monitor (preferably a video monitor)
2. Blackout curtains
3. A comfortable crib and white noise machine
4. Diapers (if the child is not old enough to start potty training)
5. A pacifier, rocker, etc.

All these items are very helpful during sleep training.

The baby monitor enables you know what's going on with the baby before you get to the room. The audio monitor lets you know if the baby is crying and whether he needs attention. The video monitor is even better as it lets you watch the baby without being present. Blackout curtains help to block bright lights, especially during the day. It reduces the amount of light in the room and helps the baby feel comfortable. You should also get a comfortable crib or rocker for your baby. No items should be placed in the crib apart from the mattress.

One of the most important things you need to do is to create a perfect environment. The area should be free from loud sounds and bright lights. Give the baby warm baths and massages before bedtime to help her relax.

PART TWO

***

FIRST STEPS

CHAPTER ONE

***

STEPS TO TAKE FOR SUCCESSFUL SLEEP TRAINING

*I*n this section, we'll take you through the important steps to take for sleep training to be successful.

There are some scenarios you are most likely to encounter during sleep training and it is important that you know how to go about them. First, you should have an open mind about the process; you shouldn't be one-dimensional in your sleep training methods. Each baby is unique, so some methods might need slight adjustments or modification based on your baby's temperament.

Before you start sleep training, make sure your baby is ready, and you also. It doesn't make sense to start at a period when you will be very busy and may not have someone to help you out. Also, if your baby has trouble sleeping through the night and also during the daytime, you can check for any health issues, and with a clean bill of health, you can then start sleep training. Meanwhile, you shouldn't forget to get the necessary sleep training items for your baby like the baby monitor, blackout curtains, pacifiers, crib, etc. Above all, you should be mentally prepared for possible sleepless nights and having to attend to the baby at various times. With the right methods and consistency, the process will be over before you know it.

What Should You Do When Your Baby Wakes Up?

This is a question that comes frequently to the mind of many parents. What should they do when the child wakes up, especially in the night? Many parents are split between leaving the child to cry it out, go back to sleep himself, or to comfort him and get the child back to sleep. We'll explain the best thing to do in this situation which is convenient for both you and the baby.

To know the right thing to do when your baby wakes up, it is important to try to determine why the baby is up. You should study your baby to know his sleeping habits and what may cause sleep disturbances. Getting a baby monitor is strongly advised as it helps to view or hear the baby without needing to come to the room. This will help you determine the next action to take. Sometimes, the baby make wake up at random times during sleep for no specific reason, especially if he hasn't gone into a deep sleep. This occurs in adults as well. Usually, the baby will go back to sleep on his own within seconds or a few minutes without any intervention. In cases such as this, the baby doesn't cry much or even cry at all. In this situation, the best thing to do is to leave the baby for a while, especially if he isn't crying or visibly distressed, to see if he will go back to sleep on his own. A baby monitor will enable you to see this properly without needing to attend to the baby.

Lifting the baby or coming into the room might further disturb the baby's sleep. Only do this if the baby doesn't go back to sleep within a few minutes or is starting to get uncomfortable. According to research, babies will wake up naturally two to six times each night.

At times, you may need to lift the baby and gently rock him to sleep if he is used to that. Babies may be scared at times if they wake up alone or in a place different from where they were before they slept. In this case you may need to soothe her until she goes back to sleep. In other cases, the baby might be hungry, feeling hot or cold, or generally uncomfortable.

Your Baby's Reflexes: To Swaddle or Not?

Swaddling refers to wrapping the baby in blankets or other clothing to calm him and to restrict his movements. Though swaddling when done correctly can help to soothe your baby, it also comes with some risks if done incorrectly. According to the American Academy of Pediatrics, swaddling can increase the risk of Sudden Infant Death Syndrome (SIDS) when done with the baby lying on their stomach, or if the baby rolls onto their stomach during sleep. Some studies also suggest swaddling may pose some other health risks such as affected arousal thresholds and lower respiratory tract infection, though these have not been fully confirmed.

Swaddling prevents babies from waking themselves up with what is known as the **Moro reflex**. The Moro reflex is a reflex process present in babies up to 3 to 4 months of age. It involves three stages. First, the baby spreads out her arms, then starts to pull them back in. This stage is often followed by crying. In other words, the processes are *abduction, adduction, and crying.* Swaddling helps to keep the baby's limbs very close to prevent these movements.

Swaddling must, however, be **done with the utmost care**. If you wrap the baby loosely, he might kick the blanket off easily. If you use too much cloth, the baby's temperature might increase above the normal levels, which will eventually lead to crying. The baby is also at the risk of choking if the cloth is loose, so it's important to make sure the baby is secured properly. Also, the blankets should have a little space at the legs to prevent hip dysplasia and to ensure proper hip development. There are some modern swaddles which have been designed with all these in mind and are safe for your baby.

Do not wrap the baby loosely,
and in too much cloth

If the baby is old enough to **roll over**, the swaddle should be changed to a **light covering** which allows for more movement. Swaddling offers some benefits but comes with some risk, so it is not advisable for long-term practice.

Putting Your Baby Into The Crib

Crib training is also part of sleep training. According to the American Academy of Pediatrics, babies should sleep in the same room but not **in the same bed as their parents** for the first six months and up to a year. Most newborns will prefer to sleep in your arms or close to you rather than in a crib, so it is necessary that you select the right crib for your baby and let him get familiar with it.

If the baby sleeps in your arms all the time, she might not get used to sleeping in the crib as she will prefer the warmth and comfort of your arms. This is why you should make the crib as comfortable as possible. To start with, you can let the baby doze off in your arms. As soon as she is drifting to sleep, you can place her gently into the crib. For starters, the crib should be placed in your room or any other room the child is familiar with. After that, you should then create a consistent bedtime routine for your baby which should end by you placing her in the crib.

For safety purposes, you shouldn't place *toys, pillows, or loose blankets* in the crib together with your baby, to prevent suffocation. If the baby is still little, he can be swaddled, but properly to give additional comfort. The baby should always sleep on his back when in the crib. If the baby is younger than four months and begins to fuss while in the crib, pick him up and soothe him until he calms down. Do this repeatedly until he falls asleep. For older babies, you can keep a little distance. If he starts to fuss in the crib, you can calm him down verbally or gently rub him until he falls asleep completely. You'll need to comfort the baby frequently at the start but can then reduce the contact as time goes on to enable him sleep independently.

This process requires consistency; however, once the baby has started sleeping in the crib, you shouldn't go back to the bassinet or any other place.

How to Lull Your Baby to Sleep

Most times, you need to create some white noise to get your baby to sleep, especially if you are just starting sleep training. Contrary to what most people believe, newborns need some kind of noise to help them sleep. Total silence is strange for the baby. According to research, the baby hears sounds equivalent to that of a vacuum cleaner while in the womb. They are still accustomed to that for the first few months so there is the need for a calming background noise to help them sleep.

If your baby experiences discomfort during sleep or any other sleep disturbance, you can lift her up by the side and whisper *"shhhh."* If she is crying, make sure the *"shush"* is almost as loud as her cry. Do this until she goes back to sleep. There are some other white noise sounds you can play while your baby is asleep. There are two types of white noise: high frequency and low frequency. Alarm sounds, pagers, and sirens are all high-frequency sounds, while train sounds, cars, rumbling, etc. are low-frequency sounds which help to soothe your baby better. The baby is more used to the low frequency sounds in the womb, which is filled with fluid which filters out the high-frequency sounds. Lulling can also be accompanied with slow movements.

The Art of Rocking a Baby

Rocking or other gentle movements are another way to get your child to sleep. They are among the most common ways of comforting babies when they are upset or if they experience a sleep disturbance. While in the womb, babies are used to gentle movements so this can help them calm down when they are upset. Rocking can also be done with baby rockers and swings as the baby grows older. Rocking can easily become a bedtime routine for the baby as they'll expect to be rocked anytime they need to go to sleep. Rocking as a general term covers patting, cuddling, walking around, jiggling, swaying, car rides, and using an electric baby swing.

Though rocking is an effective method of getting your baby to sleep, over time, it may become unreliable. It's advised to use other techniques also as the baby grows older. In newborns who are very sensitive to movement, you might need to rock them constantly to get them to sleep. When they are put down into the crib or bassinet, they might detect your absence and will wake up. In this case, you might need to use a hammock or swing to help your baby get enough sleep. Keep in mind that babies under three months will wake up many times, so they need additional help in getting the recommended hours of sleep each day.

Once you have started rocking your baby, gradually reduce the amount and frequency once he begins to fall asleep. Let the baby fall asleep totally on the bed rather than on you.

Whenever you suspect that your child is about to rouse, rock him slightly to help him get back to sleep. Babies over five months old will wake naturally between four to six times in a night. To sleep through the night, they need to reset the sleep stages many times before completing the sleep cycle. **The longer they are rocked to sleep, the more often they will wake during the night.**

Rocking sounds very simple but in practice requires coordination and consistency, or the opposite of what you want will happen instead. To rock a baby properly, you need to make gentle, regular sideways movements. If you have problems with maintaining a steady movement, you can play a slow song and rock her to the beat. You should also pay attention to the baby and take note of which rhythm keeps her calm. Once you get a rhythm which does this, be consistent with it until she starts to fall asleep. There is no single position that works for every baby. Some prefer to be rocked face down while others prefer a sideways motion. It all depends on what works for your baby.

Another thing to note when rocking the baby is that you should keep the child close to your body whenever you are rocking him so as not to trigger his Moro reflex. The baby will feel more comfortable when close to your body. He'll also feel safe and warm and will go to sleep quicker than when he feels alone. This is an advantage that comes with rocking your baby yourself rather than using swings and rockers. Remember, only rock your child until he becomes sleepy, not until he falls asleep totally. This will prevent the habit of needing your help to get to sleep.

*Only rock your child until he
becomes sleepy*

Baby Pacifier: Pros and Cons

Newborns generally have a sucking reflex and will suck their thumbs and any objects they can fit into their mouth. This gives them a soothing and calming effect. It is also used in weaning the baby. Most parents prefer their babies to suck on pacifiers instead of their fingers or other objects. Like most baby care objects, pacifiers have advantages and disadvantages.

Pros

1. They help to soothe fussy babies

Pacifiers help to calm uncomfortable babies as it soothes their sucking reflex. Babies who have just been weaned or who are still in the process might wake up during sleep expecting to suck on something. They might end up frustrated when there is nothing available. Pacifiers will help to calm them down. Even babies who have a full stomach might show this sucking reflex, so pacifiers help to keep them happy.

2. They help to distract babies for a while

Sometimes your baby might wake up from sleep due to some unknown or inconsequential reason and have a hard time going back to sleep. Pacifiers can be used to distract her for some time before she goes back to sleep. Also, they can be used in a variety of other situations where you need to keep her busy.

3. They can help babies relieve ear pain during a flight

As an airplane ascends, the change in air pressure causes a slight pain or discomfort in the ears. Most adults are able to relieve this pressure by popping their ears; however, babies can't. They can only relieve this pressure by sucking. A pacifier will help in this case.

4. They reduces the risk of sudden infant death syndrome (SIDS)

According to some researchers, sucking on a pacifier during naps or at nighttime can reduce the risk of sudden infant death syndrome in babies. Though the research isn't clear on how it works, some researchers agree that sucking on pacifiers can help reduce the risks of SIDS.

5. They encourage self-soothing in babies

Pacifiers help babies calm and relax themselves and feel comfortable.

Pacifiers offer some possible disadvantages, which include:

1. They may cause problems with breastfeeding

Using pacifiers might affect breastfeeding negatively. Babies can tell the difference between sucking on a breast and sucking on a pacifier. This can therefore shorten breastfeeding periods and their frequency. This is why you should defer pacifier use until some weeks after your baby is born so that he does not develop a preference to pacifiers over breastfeeding.

2. Your baby might become "addicted" to the pacifier

Your baby may become so used to the pacifier that she'll start to cry whenever she is without it. If the pacifier falls out during naps or during the night and your baby wakes up without it, she may begin to fuss and cry and you'll have to spend extra time getting her to sleep again.

3. Prolonged use can cause tooth problems

Ordinarily, using pacifiers for some months or a few years won't cause permanent problems; however, using them over a long period might affect your baby's tooth development. Their teeth might become misaligned or slanted with long-term use, especially after two years old.

4. Ear infections

According to a research, babies who suck on pacifiers have a higher chance of getting ear infections than children who do not.

If you decide to use pacifiers for your baby, there are some helpful tips which could be highly beneficial. First, **do not give your baby a pacifier that has a cord attached to it. This can strangle the baby if left unchecked**. Also, you should make sure the pacifier is the right size for your baby's mouth. It shouldn't be too big or too small. If you have more than one baby, they shouldn't share a pacifier. Each baby should have their own, which should be kept clean at all times to prevent infection.

When buying a pacifier, make sure you choose one that has ventilation holes in it to reduce the risk of choking. Also, do not add sweet or sugary substances to the pacifier to persuade your baby to hold on to it. It will cause a sugar addiction in the long run and might affect your baby's teeth. Pacifiers shouldn't be used for an extremely long period; you should wean your baby off it when it is obvious he no longer needs it. You can limit the use slowly until he eventually stops using it at all.

Rockers and Bouncers: Pros and Cons

If you want to keep your baby calm or entertained while you attend to other things, baby rockers can be the best option for you. Lifting your newborn and rocking him yourself might be easy at first, but as the baby grows bigger, the process can become tiring and monotonous. Your baby may also start to take longer to fall asleep and you might not have the patience to rock him gently until he falls asleep. Most parents prefer rockers and bouncers to do this job. Most baby rockers have toys or objects attached to the frame which the baby can play with to pass the time or until he falls asleep.

A baby bouncer is a seat that responds to the baby's movement and bounces up and down with her kicks. In most, the baby will be placed in a semi-upright position and strapped to the seat. As the baby tries to move, the bouncer also moves up and down, giving a calming effect. There are some models that do more than this; some vibrate with each movement while some play music or have other features.

Bouncers and rockers both serve more than one purpose: they help to entertain your baby, calm him down, and also help him fall asleep faster. They offer many advantages, but there are some drawbacks you should know about before purchasing one for your baby. These pros and cons will be explained below.

Advantages

1. Bouncers and rockers help to reduce the baby's falling reflex as they help develop the baby's sense of balance. The baby eventually learns to control the tempo of the bouncing or rocking motions.

2. They help to entertain babies and keep them calm. Bouncers and rockers eliminate the need for you to attend to your baby all the time, as the baby can entertain herself by bouncing up and down.

3. Bouncers and rockers help to improve your baby's sleep. While in the womb, babies get used to rocking motions and after they are born, these gentle movements help to calm then down and initiate sleep.

4. Baby jumpers and bouncers can help strengthen the baby's leg muscles. As the baby pushes up in the bouncer or jumper, he exercises his leg muscles, which helps to prepare them for when he'll start to crawl and walk.

Disadvantages

1. Baby bouncers put babies at the risk of sustaining neck injuries and some other injuries. As the baby is still developing, the neck muscles and other core muscles still lack the strength to handle any force exerted from the head, as their head contains a significant portion of their body weight. This can put the baby at the risk of sustaining neck and body injuries, especially if she is placed at a wrong position.

2. Bouncers also puts the baby at the risk of experiencing breathing difficulties. If the baby gets into a wrong position due to the bouncer's motion, he might not be able to breathe properly and won't be able to adjust himself.

3. The baby might develop **positional plagiocephaly.** This is known as a situation where a flat spot develops on the baby's head due to lying in the same position for a long period of time. The baby's bones are still soft and are easily affected by posture and pressure.

4. The baby is at the risk of falling from an unsecured bouncer. Also, some types of bouncers may put the baby at the risk of strangulation, especially doorway jumpers.

When using bouncers for your baby, make sure you check on them very frequently. Check if they are in a safe position and lift them out of the bouncer once in a while to change their position. You should only get bouncers and rockers that have enough safety straps and harnesses, although these straps should not also pose a risk for your baby. The bouncer should not be placed on a raised or uneven surface to prevent the risk of falling.

Though bouncers and rockers are fun for babies, you should limit their use. Ensure they only use them for a certain number of minutes at a time. If the baby is grown enough, he should be placed on the floor periodically to help improve his motor skills. Once the baby is capable of making a wide range of motions, it is advisable to ditch the bouncer as it gradually becomes **unsafe for a very active baby**.

Practical Steps on Sleep Training Methods

Regardless of the sleep training method you want to use, there are some practical steps common to them all which you can take. These will be listed below.

1. Create a proper sleep environment first

Before you even try to get your baby to sleep, the room must be ready. The lights dimmed, the curtains drawn down, and the baby's crib well prepared.

2. Prepare the baby for bedtime or naptime

Depending on your baby, there are some bedtime routines you can incorporate into the sleep training process. It can either be a massage, a warm bath, exercise, or another safe activity that can calm your baby down. You should experiment to see what works for your baby's temperament, as some bedtime routines might achieve the opposite effect. For example, a warm bath can make some babies even more excited.

3. Swaddle or Rock the Baby

You'll need to help the child soothe himself first if he hasn't developed self-soothing yet. For babies young enough, you can swaddle or gently rock and lull them until they begin to fall asleep.

4. Place the child in the crib or bassinet

After the child has started falling asleep, place her in the crib or wherever she sleeps each night—not beside you, however. The crib should not contain any loose objects or toys, and should be made as comfortable as possible.

5. Stay for some minutes

In the early stages of sleep training, your child might experience early sleep disturbances. You can stay for a few minutes to help him get back to sleep in case he wakes up. You can leave the room once he falls asleep totally.

CHAPTER TWO

✷✷✷

HOW YOUR BABY'S TEMPERAMENT AFFECTS SLEEP

There have been a number of studies on how babies' temperaments affect their sleep. In this chapter, you'll learn the possible baby temperaments and how to suit your baby's needs by adjusting bedtime routines to fit their temperament. It is very important to know your baby's temperament and to factor it in your sleep training methods. If not, your methods might achieve the opposite effect of what you desire. For example, some bedtime routines might make your baby more active and less eager to sleep if he is the very active type, whereas it may work well for babies with gentle temperaments. Some babies have self-soothing temperaments and can go to sleep without your help most times while some do not.

What is Your Baby's Temperament?

Temperament generally refers to the overall category of emotional reactions and responses to the environment. In babies, it has been discovered that the general temperament and sleep temperament can both affect sleep. There are two types of sleep temperaments, according to research: **self-soothers and signalers**. A number of psychiatrists believe there are three general types of baby temperaments. This is quite different from the sleep temperaments mentioned in previous lines. This has to do with their general behavior apart from their sleeping habits. We'll go through the general baby temperaments first and then the sleep temperaments after.

According to psychiatrists, there are three basic types or clusters of baby temperaments, or behavioral styles exhibited by babies. This includes how active they are, how social they are, and their natural way of responding. The three temperaments are: **The Easy Child, The Difficult Child,** and **The Slow to Warm Up Child.** You can easily categorize your child into one of these groups as you watch his expressions and daily patterns.

The easy child is at most times in a positive mood and can easily adapt to new experiences. Such a child can easily follow regular routines right from infancy. Studies have shown that around 40 percent of children are in this category. The easy child has regular sleeping and toileting habits, a moderate to high energy level and can approach new people and situations quite easily. The easy child has low to moderate reactions to pleasant and unpleasant experiences. Babies who belong to this category are quite easy to sleep train, though you have to employ methods which suit their activity levels.

The difficult child is the opposite of the easy child. Children in this category are more likely to react negatively to new experiences and they also cry frequently. The difficult child has a high level of energy but is reluctant to embrace new situations and people. Such children show visible expressions whenever they are frustrated, angry, or happy.

The slow to warm up child has low activity levels, their mood intensity is also low, and they are very reluctant to encounter new situations and people.

There are two sleep temperaments, and your baby might fall under either. Though babies wake up between five to seven times during the night, babies who are self-soothers do not usually need help in going back to sleep. They are able to do this on their own through the night. Self-soothers also go to sleep easily when it's bedtime than babies who aren't. They can sleep for longer periods and are able to sleep through the night faster than babies with the other sleep temperament.

The other type of babies based on their sleep temperament are signalers. These type of babies take longer to go to sleep and they also learn self-soothing later than the self-soothing babies. Babies in this category will take longer to fall asleep and if they wake during the night, they'll have a hard time going back to sleep. We'll go through how to identify your baby's temperament in the next section.

Identifying Your Baby's Temperament

As a parent, you'll need to identify your baby's temperament which will help you choose the right sleep training methods for him. There are markers or peculiarities you can look out for to determine the category under which your baby falls in. We'll examine the more peculiar features of the two sleep temperaments below.

To determine if your baby is a signaler, there are some sleep habits you need to check out for. First, does she wake up at regular times each night? Does she only calm down if she sees you coming into the room when she's crying? If so, then your baby is certainly a signaler. These are not the only features to check out for, but they are the easiest ones to notice. There are other features of signalers we've mentioned in the previous section such as taking a long time to fall asleep or waking up many times during the night.

To determine whether your baby falls under the category of self-soothers, these are things to watch for: Does your child go back to sleep easily after waking up? Does he practice self-soothing? Can he sleep for long periods at a stretch? These are among the questions you should answer to help you know your baby's category. Self-soothers are usually content with using pacifiers or sucking their thumb to soothe themselves. If your baby does this often, then he might be a self-soother.

Some methods which work for babies of other temperaments might not work if they aren't suitable for your baby's temperament. Things such as a warm bath can have different effects on babies. Some babies will get tired when it's close to bedtime and will only need something to relax them further before they go to sleep. Rocking or massaging such babies is usually enough to get them to sleep. Other babies might actually need to burn their excess energy before going to sleep. All you need to do is just to pay attention to your baby to know what the best option is for her.

Scientific Research on Sleep Temperaments

According to Dr. Elizabeth Super, a pediatrician and children's sleep specialist at the Children's Hospital in Portland, Oregon, despite the baby's natural sleep temperaments, sleep skills are actually a learned behavior and as they grow up, they will need to learn and adjust their sleep temperament to help them sleep independently. If your baby isn't a self-soother, it doesn't mean that he won't be able to sleep through the night eventually without your help.

According to research conducted by Kataria, Swanson & Trevathan in 1987, some individual differences in the sleep development and the course of the maturation of sleeping habits have been linked to sleep temperaments. This means there are some natural peculiarities which may affect your child's sleep development. In another study, it was discovered that parental practices also affect the development of sleep self-regulation. Practices such as bedtime routine consistency, sleep independence training and the gradual reduction of parental proximity during sleep all influence the development of sleep self-regulation in babies.

According to O'Connor et al, in research conducted in 2007, "Temperamental style is modified by the attachment relationship and other socializing experiences that may expand or suppress predisposing psychological experiences." In simpler terms, this means your child's sleep temperament can be modified by some bedtime practices which can either help to expand favorable natural sleep habits, such as in self-soothing babies, or to restrict undesirable natural sleep habits, such as in signalers.

What Type of Sleep Training is Better For You?

It may get confusing seeing different sleep training methods, with people telling you they all work. However, it shouldn't be so difficult for you to choose one that will works for your baby and is also convenient for you. Any sleep training method you choose must be recommended by pediatricians and must be suitable for your baby's temperament. **When trying out a sleep training method, make sure you choose one you can easily stick with.** For example, some methods which strictly encourage self-soothing right from the start of the training might get uncomfortable for you and the other members of your household, especially if the baby starts crying at night.

There are some other factors you should consider before choosing any sleep training methods such as age, personal beliefs, and your child's sleep patterns. Some methods might also need adjustments based on your baby and your own schedule. In all, choose a method that's safe for your baby and be consistent with it.

CHAPTER THREE

***

SLEEP AND FEEDING

Feeding Your Baby

Hunger is among the common reasons babies wake up during the night or during naps, and you have to factor in your baby's feeding schedule during sleep training if you don't want to lengthen the process. Naturally, babies need to eat during the night as well as throughout the day, especially during the first few months. The first thing you need to do is to take note of your baby's feeding patterns to help you develop a feeding schedule. At a point, the baby will be developed enough to stop night feeding and will start to develop noticeable feeding patterns. They get enough calories during the day to last for five to six hours in the night.

A common tactic parents use is to feed the child to sleep. While this is beneficial in the first three to four months, as babies at that age need to eat every few hours, it can become an issue after the first few months. It might become the only way for you to get your child to sleep once it becomes a habit.

Should You Feed the Baby on Demand Or on Schedule?

This is a question on the minds of many parents: should they feed the child randomly or should they set a feeding schedule? This all **depends on how old the baby is**. At a point, you'll have to stop feeding the child at night if you want him to sleep through the night, but before that, there are some times you'll need to feed on demand. According to researchers, during the **first three months, babies do not develop any self-soothing abilities yet and they may need to eat every few hours.** At this stage, they have an irregular sleep-wake cycle, so it is better to feed them on demand.

Feeding on a schedule might not work during the first three months as the baby may not be hungry during the scheduled periods, or may need to eat before the scheduled periods. This can be chaotic for both you and the baby, so the best thing to do at this stage is to feed the baby on demand. However, though the baby's feeding and sleep schedules are irregular at this age, it can still be possible to get an idea of his future patterns. Breastfed newborns typically need to eat every two to three hours, so you should be able to get an idea of when he needs to feed. Gradually, he will start to develop predictable feeding patterns. Before this, you can feed the baby whenever he is hungry, but remember, this should only go on for the first few months.

Feeding on demand has some benefits for newborns and mothers alike. First, it ensures the baby gets enough nutrients to develop properly. Also, for breastfeeding mothers, it helps to ensure a steady milk flow. The more you feed the baby, the more milk you produce. It also allows for proper bonding between the mother and the child.

Scheduled feedings are necessary when the **baby is above four months**. To do this, you schedule convenient feeding periods for your baby. Though the feeding periods will be set by you, it should also be close to your baby's natural feeding schedule. Scheduled feeding is particularly important if you need to stop nighttime feeding for your baby. Eating at night might become a habit for him if you do not introduce scheduled feeding. Once the baby is developed to a stage, there will be no need to feed him at night as he is now able to sleep four up to six hours without feeding. The feeding periods are initiated by you and not your baby. You can set alarms to help remind you when it's time to feed. The baby should be close to bedtime but there should be other consistent bedtime routines also.

Scheduled feeding is easier for you as a parent than on-demand feeding. This is because there will be specific feeding periods and you do not have to get up at random times to feed your baby. For scheduled feeding, you shouldn't quit night feeding cold turkey. Rather, reduce the frequency gradually until it stops eventually. This is to give the baby enough time to adjust and to **gradually develop their self-soothing abilities**. The scheduled feeding periods shouldn't interfere with the child's sleep. If the baby is asleep, it might be better to wait until he rouses until you feed him. In scheduled feeding, there are some important things you should take note of.

First, if you are breastfeeding, scheduled feeding might affect your milk supply. This is why you should make the feedings as frequent as possible. Also, your baby's development will be affected if he doesn't get enough food. It may be hard for you to determine if the baby is full or not but you can check for signs such as when the baby releases repeatedly during breastfeeding. There will be growth spurts during the baby's development, so you should take note of this too. The baby will need to feed more times than usual during this period.

Overall, scheduled feeding is easier for you as a parent than on-demand feeding. However, you should make sure your child is above three months before you practice this.

Why It Is Important to Stick to the Schedule

As soon as your baby starts to develop a natural feeding pattern, it is important to create a feeding schedule which must be consistent. It is important to follow the feeding schedule because inconsistency will cause problems with sleep training. Your baby might wake up hungry at random times when you might not be prepared if you do not follow the feeding schedule. This will disrupt both the baby's sleep and yours.

Also, following the sleep schedule also helps to promote proper feeding habits. When timed with the baby's natural feeding pattern, a consistent feeding schedule will ensure the baby gets enough calories needed to develop.

Basics and Tips When Breastfeeding

Breastfeeding can help your child calm down during sleep training. It is also an opportunity for you to bond with your baby. According to researchers, sucking helps to release a hormone called cholecystokinin in both babies and mothers, which induces a sleepy feeling. For babies who are above four months or old enough to sleep through the night without feeding, it is necessary to feed them at regular times, especially when it's close to bedtime. Make sure your baby gets enough milk before he goes to sleep each night to prevent sleep disturbances.

If your baby isn't able to sleep through the night yet, especially for babies under four months, nighttime breastfeeding is necessary. If the baby wakes up during the night, nurse him and soothe him until he goes back to sleep. Babies under four months might need to be breastfed several times each night, as breast milk is digested very fast. As the baby develops, you can reduce nighttime breastfeeding gradually until it stops completely. However, breastfeeding can be a part of your baby's bedtime routine. It is one of the easiest ways to get your baby to sleep at bedtime.

Basics and Tips When Bottle-feeding

If you opt for bottle-feeding your baby, there are some helpful tips you should read to help you with feeding during the sleep training process. Bottle-feeding during sleep training is easier, especially for working parents. According to childcare specialists, breast-fed infants are more likely to wake up at night than bottle-fed infants, especially if the baby is being fed with baby formula. Feeding the baby is easier during sleep training as if you are not available, another member of your household can help you feed the baby, once there is a supply of breast milk for the baby.

When bottle-feeding your baby, either or demand or on schedule, always make sure you express enough milk in a bottle which should be readily available. It should be kept safely in a refrigerator. You also shouldn't leave the bottle alone with your baby as it can be dangerous. The feeding periods should also be different if you are feeding your baby with formula. Formula takes about four hours to digest, as compared to two hours for breastmilk. You should feed the baby a few minutes or hours before bedtime and after you do so, burp him, to help dispel the air swallowed during feeding.

Feeding at night: Basics and Tips

For some months, you will need to feed your baby at various times through the night. You might then be faced with the problem of how to feed your child during the night without interrupting sleep training. To solve this, there are some guidelines to follow.

First, you shouldn't wake the child up to feed him during the night, except if the child has feeding problems or is underweight. Doing this will interfere with the child's natural sleep cycles. It is best to wait for the baby to wake by himself, after which you can feed him until he goes back to sleep again. Your baby will go back to sleep easily if he wakes up by himself and is fed. During nighttime feeding, it is also advisable to dim or switch off the lights. This will help the baby get back to sleep right after feeding. If not, you might be left with an active baby and you'll then need to calm him down first after feeding him.

Also, keep the noise levels down when feeding your baby at night. Your voice alone might be enough to keep him active and stimulated. With the noise levels down, it'll be easier for him to get back to sleep after feeding. Remember to burp your baby after each feeding session.

CHAPTER FOUR

***

SLEEP TRAINING METHODS

*I*n this chapter, we'll go through the popular sleep training methods, which include the no-cry method, the cry-it-out-method, the chair method, the Ferber method, the wake and sleep technique, and the fading method.

The No-cry Method

This sleep training approach is the opposite of the cry-it-out method. Advocates of this method encourage offering comfort as soon as a baby starts to cry or fuss. Though this method might take more time to work than some sleep training methods, the approach is gentler than the cry-it-out method. However, it requires dedication, as you have to be always available for your baby. This is more suited to stay-at-home parents or parents who can pay **round-the-clock** attention to their baby. It also requires lots of soothing as you'll have to calm the baby down every single time he starts to cry.

Though this method is very comfortable for the baby, it has some downsides. First, it doesn't encourage self-soothing. Your baby will take a longer time before he starts to sleep through the night independently. She will simply cry for most reasons once she knows you are always available. Also, this approach isn't comfortable for most parents, as you'll have to attend to your child many times during the day and at night. You'll have to be prepared to lose a lot of sleep with this method.

The Cry-it-out Method

This method is one of the most controversial sleep training methods. It involves allowing the baby to simply cry without intervening until they are able to soothe themselves. There are variants of this method, such as the Ferber method. The main advantage of this method is that it promotes self-soothing in babies. The baby will learn to soothe himself faster than in most sleep training methods. However, critics have said that this method can cause some psychological damage to your baby. It can also be inconvenient for parents. Having to listen to your child cry can be frustrating and heartbreaking.

The Chair Method

In this method, as the name implies, the parent has to sit close to the crib but without maintaining contact with the baby.

As the baby falls asleep, the parent then moves farther away from the crib until the baby falls asleep totally.

The aim of this method is not to help the baby fall asleep; it is only to make the baby aware of your presence.

This method is a bit better for parents than the cry-it-out method as the baby might not cry for long when he knows you are close. It isn't as fast as the cry-it-out approach, however.

The Ferber Method

This method is a variant of the cry-it-out approach and was developed by a pediatrician named Dr. Richard Ferber. Often mistaken for the cry-it-out approach, this method involves making sure the baby is drowsy before placing him in the crib and then leaving the room. If the baby starts crying, the parent then waits for some minutes before attending to the baby. The number of minutes will then increase gradually as the days go by, for example, from 5 minutes, to 10 minutes, and so on. This technique helps to prevent a long time of crying by the baby. It is a more comfortable approach than the cry-it-out method, though slower.

If you prefer the Ferber method, there are some steps to take to make sure sleep training is successful. First, make sure the necessary bedtime routines are performed first to make sure the baby is ready for bed. It could be a warm massage, a warm bath, or any other bedtime activity suitable for your baby. After that, prepare the room and the crib, and rock or gently swing the baby until he becomes drowsy.

Once the baby becomes **drowsy but not totally asleep**, place him in the crib and leave the room. If the child starts to cry or fuss after you've left, wait for a certain number of minutes before going in to soothe him. You can start with two minutes for a baby new to sleep training. As the baby gradually learns to self-soothe, you can then increase the number of minutes you wait for before coming in. This will continue until the baby learns how to self-soothe.

The Wake and Sleep Technique

This method involves waking the child up from sleep to let them fall asleep independently. The parent can then assist the baby a little bit to help him get back to sleep. This method, along with the cry-it out approach, is part of the fastest methods to help your child learn self-soothing. However, though the method is fast, it is very uncomfortable for the baby and it can affect the child's natural sleep cycle.

The method can also lead to sleep deprivation in babies and even in parents, as you have to wake the child up from sleep at intervals. The child may also not go through the complete sleep stages before waking up. Studies have also shown that sleep disturbances or irregular sleep can affect hormone release and metabolism.

The wake and sleep method starts like most methods. Help the child get to sleep after the necessary bedtime routines, after which you'll put the child in the crib or bassinet. After a certain number of minutes or hours, like every two hours during nighttime, gently move the child until he wakes up, and wait for him to go back to sleep again. If the child doesn't get back to sleep after a short while, you can then help him get back to sleep. Gradually, the child will learn to self soothe and will need little to no help in getting back to sleep.

The Fading Method

This method involves gradually diminishing the soothing techniques you use on your baby. It involves reducing the amount of time spent helping the baby sleep until the baby can self-soothe. This gives enough time for the baby to learn how to soothe himself. It is very convenient for both the parent and the baby, though it might take some time. The main advantage of this method is that it gives the baby sufficient time to learn how to soothe himself properly, but it is also comfortable for the baby and the parent or caregiver.

This method has some drawbacks, however. First, it might lead to a prolonged sleep training process as you'll need enough time to help your baby learn to self-soothe. It also requires dedication and consistency and may not be suitable for working parents.

The Type That Suits You Best

We've listed the popular sleep training methods along with their downsides. Depending on your schedule and tolerance, you can select one which will be convenient for you and your baby. The fading method seems to be the most balanced. It prevents your baby from crying unnecessarily while giving him the time to develop self-soothing abilities. Regardless, you should choose a method that won't be stressful for both you and the baby. One thing you should note is that babies are different. One method will not work for every baby, so you can adopt and modify the method of your choice to suit your baby's temperament. You can also pick and combine aspects of different methods to get the best results.

Myths Around Sleep Training Methods

Here are some popular myths about sleep training methods:

1. The cry-it-out method will make your child hate you

Research has shown that using the cry-it-out approach does not negatively impact the bond between the child and the parent.

2. You'll have to stop holding and playing with your child

Sleep training doesn't prevent you from having a good time with your child. Fun activities can still be part of the nighttime routine.

3. Getting another room for the baby is compulsory

This myth particularly surrounds the chair and the Ferber method. However, it is not compulsory for you to get another room for the baby. You can still create a comfortable sleeping space for the baby in the same room.

4. Sleep training is done by selfish parents

Most parents who have successfully sleep trained their child have testified that it actually benefits both the child and the parent. The child develops a regular sleeping pattern and the parent has more time to rest too.

5. The baby won't have any sleep problems after sleep training

Some factors can still affect the child's sleep later on. For example, teething is very uncomfortable for babies, and it is common for them to lose a lot of sleep during this period.

What Researchers and Pediatricians Recommend

A review of 52 studies on sleep training showed that almost all sleep training methods are effective when applied consistently. Child care specialist and developer of the Ferber approach Dr. Richard Ferber recommends teaching a baby to soothe themselves by leaving the baby alone for specific periods of time. He recommends following a consistent bedtime routine to help the child develop good sleep patterns.

William Sears, a pediatrician and author of the *Baby Sleep Book* recommends a gradual approach in encouraging self-soothing. He opines that the baby should get the comfort he needs immediately to help him get to sleep as soon as possible. This is in line with the no-cry method.

Kim West, author of *The Sleep Lady's Good Night,* says **sleep training should be a gradual process.** The child should have enough time to properly develop self-soothing abilities. This research embraces the fading method.

Marc Weissbuth, a pediatrician and author, recommends influencing the child's sleep duration once the baby is above four months (the wake and sleep technique). According to him, **babies under three months** should have a free sleep schedule as they **do not have predictable sleeping patterns**

yet, but after four months, parents can help create a regular sleep schedule.

PART THREE

***

Healthy Sleep Training and Different Sleep Stages

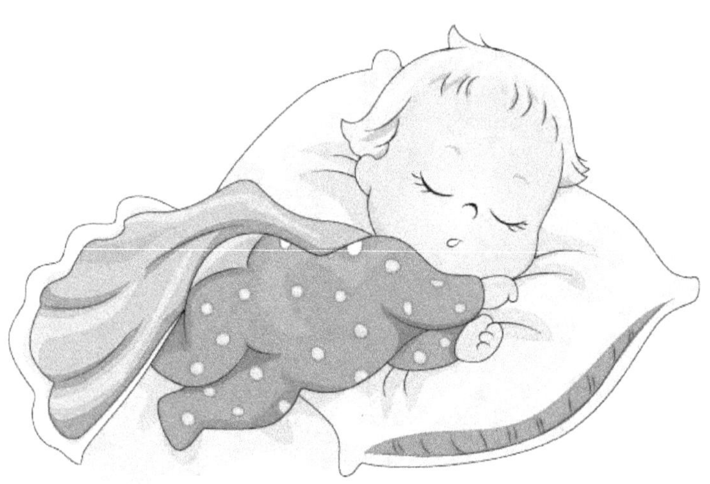

Healthy Sleep Routines For Babies Between 0-1 Month Old

though babies under four months are not ready for full sleep training, it doesn't negate the importance of maintaining a healthy bedtime routine. A healthy bedtime routine goes a long way in making the sleep training process easy when the baby is ready for it. Babies at this age should get 15-18 hours of sleep each day, according to pediatricians. Babies between 0-1 month still have irregular sleep cycles and stay awake for two to three hours at a stretch. At this stage, the baby's natural sleep schedules should be followed. You can only make sure the baby gets the recommended hours of sleep each day by maintaining a proper environment and effective sleep routines.

Newborn babies are generally inactive and will wake most times only to feed for a short time before going back to sleep. When your baby wakes up in this case, make sure he gets fed properly until he releases. The diaper should also be changed frequently to prevent irritation. After feeding, you can swaddle the baby or make gentle sideways movements. Whichever one you prefer, make sure the room is good enough and the baby is also kept warm to help him sleep comfortably. At this age, the best thing is to keep your child close to you as they still require much body contact. Once the baby falls asleep, you can then place him gently into the crib or bassinet.

You can also help reinforce the baby's natural sleep and wake cycles by stimulating the child when she is awake and helping her sleep when she needs to. To do this, you can play with the child or introduce more light in the room for a few minutes to two hours whenever she is awake. If you then notice the child needs some sleep, help her get comfortable and soothe her until she falls asleep. The main difference in the temperament of babies between 0-1 month old is that some babies may cry a bit more than others and may take a longer time to get to sleep. Regardless, babies around this age are mostly asleep for the most part of the day.

The main problem that occurs during this age is the issue of sleep disturbance, and the most common reason is that the baby is hungry, hot or cold, uncomfortable, or wet. Their natural sleep rhythms are still developing so it's common for them to wake up at intervals. All you have to do is to make sure the baby is as comfortable as possible.

For newborns, on-demand feeding seems to be the best feeding option to make sure your baby gets enough food. The baby's sleep and wake patterns are still irregular at this stage so the feeding schedule shouldn't follow a strict pattern for now.

Healthy Sleep Routines For Babies Between 1-2 Months Old

Babies between one to two months old should sleep for fifteen to seventeen hours each day. They should sleep for around six to seven hours during the day in the form of three to four naps and around eight hours at night. Babies this age still need to be fed every two to four hours. Healthy babies do not usually need to be woken up to be fed at this age. The baby's circadian rhythm is still underdeveloped so they'll wake up many times during daytime and nighttime to be fed.

Babies under four months are still not fully ready for sleep training, but you can help them maintain a healthy sleep routine until they are ready to develop their self-soothing abilities. At two months old, a baby starts to become aware of its surroundings. They start becoming a little bit active and might need a warm massage or a soothing bath before bedtime. Babies this age are usually awake for between 45 minutes to 2 hours at a time. Breastfed babies will need to be fed every two to four hours while formula-fed babies will need to be fed around six times per day.

At this period, you'll need to help your baby get back to sleep each time he experiences a sleep disturbance. The no-cry method is essential for babies below three months old, as they are yet to develop self-soothing. If the baby experiences a sleep disturbance, gently soothe her until she goes back to sleep. The baby should always sleep on her back as other positions can cause breathing problems and increased risk of SIDS.

As the baby is gradually developing at this age, it is important to help exercise his muscles during playtime, especially the neck muscles and the other upper body muscles. **The baby should be properly engaged whenever he is awake;** for example, the curtains can be raised and you can sing songs and talk to the baby. When it's close to bedtime, both the baby and the room should be prepared. The curtains should be drawn down, the baby should be given a warm bath or massage and then fed. After this, you can either swaddle or rock the baby gently until he falls asleep.

Healthy Sleep Routines For Babies Between 2-3 Months Old

At three months, the baby will start to develop noticeable sleep patterns and will soon be ready for sleep training. The baby will start to sleep for longer stretches ech night and will be awake for longer periods during the day. Babies at three months of age need between eleven to twelve hours of sleep each night and three to four hours during the day. The baby will start to eat less frequently during the night and will start to take a long nap followed by other short naps during the day.

At 2 to 3 months, the baby's stomach is considerably larger than it was few weeks after birth. The baby will need between 1 to 3 night feedings at this stage. Formula-fed babies will need one or possibly two night feedings. Babies also gain significant upper body strength at this period and are able to kick and stretch their legs. The baby starts to develop some motor skills so it is important to make sure she gets enough exercise and playtime activities during the day.

Although the baby isn't able to sleep through the night consistently, it is still important to establish a consistent bedtime routine. Most experts recommend feeding the baby at the beginning of the routine, followed by calming activities such as a bath or massage. At this point, you can put the baby down to sleep while drowsy but not totally asleep. The baby should be in the same room as you or the caregiver but not in the same bed.

There are some possible issues that may be encountered at this stage which might affect sleep, such as teething or sleep regression. Teething can begin in babies as early as two months and will surely affect the child's sleep as it is very uncomfortable for them. The baby might also start to have negative feelings toward bedtime. This is why **you should incorporate fun and soothing bedtime routines for your baby as early as possible**. It can be in form of bedtime stories, songs and lullabies, or warm baths. Studies have shown that reading to babies is highly beneficial. Even if you feel the baby doesn't understand, reading still helps in developing the baby's communication skills, listening skills, and overall cognitive development.

set up soothing bedtime routines: bath, stories, lullabies

Another problem commonly faced during this period is fitful sleep. Late night or midnight feeding can make babies restless. This is why it is important to make sure your baby gets enough food before bedtime to reduce the frequency of late night feedings. At this stage, the fading method is the most recommended as the child is just learning how to self-soothe.

Healthy Sleep Routines For Babies Between 3-6 Months Old

Most experts agree that babies are fully ready for sleep training between three to six months old. At this stage, the sleep patterns are quite noticeable and sleep training methods can be fully applied. Babies between 3 to 6 months are generally expected to sleep for between 10 to 15 hours each day. At this stage, the frequency of night feedings is reduced drastically and the baby starts to develop a regular sleep and wake pattern. At this stage, **the baby's temperament starts to influence his sleep patterns**. Some babies (self-soothers) need little to no help in sleeping through the night, while others (signalers) may have a hard time self-soothing. If you pay enough attention to your child's sleep and wake habits, you'll notice the type of sleep temperament he falls under.

If your child is a signaler, you'll need to make more effort to help him sleep through the night until he can self-soothe. Regardless, you should observe your child very carefully, as each baby is unique. This will help you adopt the method that suits your child's temperament. If the child isn't ready for full sleep training yet, you can reduce the intensity and try again later. Some babies might still wake up at night to feed but should be ready for night feeding before six months.

It is important to note that sleep regressions may happen even in babies who have started to sleep for long periods or through the night. Your baby might wake up during the night or during a nap and experience problems going back to sleep for various reasons. This is especially common during teething and growth spurts. The baby also has improved motor skills at this point and may roll over during sleep, thus waking himself up.

To establish healthy sleep habits, you should create a consistent and suitable bedtime routine for your baby. Always keep your baby's temperament and activity levels in mind, since some activities might lead to the opposite of what you intend to achieve if they aren't suitable for your baby. For example, playing with her or exercising her can make her more active instead of calm before bedtime if she is the very active type. Choose a convenient bedtime for your baby, likewise regular nap times. These sleep periods should be in line with your baby's natural sleep patterns. Remember, the goal is to help your child get quality sleep and the recommended amount of sleep per day.

At this stage, you should start to encourage your baby to fall asleep independently. It is advisable to wait for a few minutes to give the baby a chance to soothe himself if he has a sleep disturbance before going in to soothe him. Babies between 3-6 months should take 3-5 naps each day, between 1 to 3 hours long. The proper pattern for babies this age is the EAT-PLAY-SLEEP routine. Eating should not be the last part of the bedtime routine so as to prevent your baby from relying on feeding in order to fall asleep. If the baby doesn't seem to be tired at the programmed bedtime, you should try a warm bath, making sure the room is prepared beforehand. You should always try as much as possible to keep up with the sleep routine.

Healthy Sleep Routines For Babies Between 6-12 Months Old

At 6 to 12 months old, the baby should have been sleep trained to a decent extent. The recommend number of hours of sleep for babies 6-12 months old is between 10-14 hours each day. The number of naps is also usually reduced to two or three at most. Between 6 to 12 months, most babies are ready to sleep through the night and if not, they are ready for night weaning. There is little to no need for night feedings as the babies get enough calories to last for five to six hours each night. This usually happens between the ages of 4 and 6 months. Your baby might wake up in the night for other reasons and may have a hard time going back to sleep if he isn't able to self soothe yet. Sleep training will help to take care of this, and with time, the baby should be able to sleep for longer periods without disturbances.

For babies between 6 to 12 months old, naps need to evenly spaced to prevent bedtime problems at night. Your baby might not need three naps if he takes long naps, just two naps might be enough in some cases. Between the ages of 6 to 12 months, sleep trained babies might experiences sleep regression and disturbances due to increased cognitive and motor development. Separation anxiety also happens usually at this stage. Your baby might become upset if he wakes up during the night alone or if he wakes up just as you're about to place him in the crib. This usually stops when they are 2 years old.

One of the ways to ease separation anxiety is to create a routine, especially a bedtime routine in the case of sleep training. Extensive use of the No-cry approach can cause separation anxiety during sleep training. This is why it is necessary to let your child develop sufficient self soothing abilities by trying out some other suitable sleep training methods or by modifying a method to suit the child. It's okay to soothe your baby at times if he cries during the night, however, the visits should be short, and once the baby is drowsy again, you can leave the room.

Also, teething can be one of the factors that might affect your baby's sleep at this stage, a cold compress can help to relieve the pain temporarily. You can also use a refrigerated teether to help pacify your baby. The teether should be kept at a safe temperature however. If the pain looks to be unbearable for the baby, you can consult a doctor who might recommend some safe painkillers for your baby.

For babies 6 to 12 months old, a bedtime routine such as having a bath, playing some gentle games, dressing up the baby for bed, reading a bedtime story or singing some lullabies is very healthy for your baby. However, these activities should be done in the same order and manner each night to ensure consistent results. Also, having a consistent daily schedule at this stage is beneficial. Though the schedule doesn't have to be very rigid, it should be predictable. In some cases, your baby might be too excited to sleep at bedtime, if this continues for a while, you can prepare the baby for bed a little bit earlier than the usual time to make sure he spends the excess energy before he goes to sleep. At this stage, swaddling might no longer be necessary, the baby can transition to a wearable blanket or a sleep sack.

Healthy Sleep Routines For Babies Between 1-3 Years Old

At one to three years old, the child now has more developed communication and motor skills and are now old enough to sleep through the night without your help. However, there are some peculiar sleep issues that can be experienced at this stage. First, there may be what is commonly known as the 18 month regression. Studies have shown that up to 20 percent of children between one and three years old still wake up many times during the night. This is largely due to unhealthy sleep habits. Meanwhile, at this age, you should no longer need to rock or nurse your toddler to sleep. The child should be able to sleep independently for 11 to 14 hours each day.

Between the ages of one and two, the number of naps usually reduces to one, or two in some cases. At this age, the child is old enough to sleep with a light blanket or some safe toys. Children this age may be restless at times and your toddler may try to climb out of the crib if you aren't watchful. This is why you should make sure the child isn't able to get hold of objects he can grasp while standing in the crib, e.g curtains, window blinds, wall hangings, or pictures.

Apart from teething pain or separation anxiety, nightmares can also be one of the factors that cause sleep disturbances. To help your toddler, you can dim the lights a bit instead of shutting them off totally so that the child isn't scared if he wakes up. You can also keep a safe toy with the child or a warm blanket to make him more comfortable. At this stage, it is important to help the child maintain proper sleep habits because bad sleep habits can be difficult to change at this stage if the child is already used to these habits. There is the need for consistency and also the need to establish limits to keep your child under control. One of these limits is screen time. **Your toddler shouldn't be with screen devices just before bedtime**. These gadgets should not also be used as a tool to get your child to sleep. Also, there shouldn't be any loud noise coming from any room close to your toddler's to help your child sleep soundly.

Your toddler may also try to go against the bed time routines just to test you, especially if he has a strong temperament. You must be firm with the rules and set clear boundaries. At this stage, the cry it out approach can be the most effective sleep training method. Since your baby now has some verbal communication skills at this age, it is not necessary to attend to him every time he fusses.

Rather than letting your child play with mobile devices until he goes to sleep, **reading books should be part of the bedtime routine**. Also, toddlers need a lot of exercise and engagement to spend any excess energy they may have. A bored or restless toddler might have a hard time sleeping through the night. However, a child who has been properly engaged during the daytime will have no problems falling asleep.

Healthy Sleep Routines For Babies Between 3-5 Years Old

According to research, children between the ages of 3 to 5 need about 11 to 13 hours of sleep per day usually with a single nap of about an hour or two. Healthy sleep is very necessary at this stage for the child's growth and development as some hormones like **the growth hormone and melatonin, are released during sleep** and the immune system can also be strengthened through proper sleeping habits. By this age, the child already has normal sleep patterns.

The main sleep problems faced during this stage are night terrors and nightmares. Also, the child may refuse to sleep alone and may choose to sleep in your bed or with any other family member. Waking up during the night is very common at this stage and might be inevitable. The only difference is that some children can go back to sleep on their own while others may need your help. Sleep disturbances may also be caused by other factors such as illness, anxiety, change of environment or new activities.

One of those sleep disturbances are night terrors. Night terrors usually happen early in the night when the child is deeply asleep. The might "wake up" suddenly and his eyes might be open but he is actually asleep. One way to know this is that the child won't respond or may sleep-talk. **If your toddler has a night terror, do not try to wake him out it,** rather, gently calm him down and guide him back to sleep until he falls asleep again. In the case of nightmares, the child may have scary or unpleasant dreams which usually occur in the second part of the night when the child dreams the most. In this case, the child is actually awake and frightened and will need assurance and comfort from you. After comforting the child, you can switch on the light if the child is scared of the dark. The lights can be dimmed and left in that state to help the child go back to sleep.

Another common sleep problem in toddlers is the refusal to settle down to sleep during bedtime or not wanting to stay in bed. **You must be consistent and firm as a parent to make them stick to the bedtime routine.** The bedtime routines should also incorporate activities that are interesting but not too tasking for the child. An overtired child may have problems settling down to sleep.

As for the bedtime routine, the child should be in bed no later than 8pm. This is because toddlers are naturally ready for bed between 7:30 pm and 8pm. They also go through the deepest stage of sleep between 8pm and midnight. The bedtime routine can start with brushing the teeth, then using the toilet, wearing the pajamas, reading books/listening to stories/lullabies, followed by getting to bed. For toddlers, excessive or time consuming play should be avoided before bedtime. There should be clear rules the child should follow when it's time for bed. Also, you should be consistent with the bedtime routines especially the bedtime rituals, for example, your child may refuse to go to sleep if he hasn't heard the usual story or lullaby before bedtime.

*Toddlers are naturally ready for
bed between 7:30 pm and 8pm*

Healthy Sleep Routines For Babies 5 Years Old and Above

Children 5 years and above should get between 9 to 13 hours of sleep per day with a nap or possibly no nap. It is advisable to let your child get at least one nap each day, though. At this stage, it might not be easy to check if your child gets enough sleep, which is why you have to pay enough attention to your child's sleep habits.

What is important at this stage is to instill and maintain proper sleep habits for your child. No screentime before bedtime, TV watching stops at a particular time, and there are bedtime activities he must follow. At this stage, the child is usually tired after coming back from school and might just need only a bath before going to bed. Regardless, the child should follow the bedtime routines you have set before going to bed.

PART FOUR

***

SLEEP DISORDERS, THEIR CAUSES AND TREATMENT

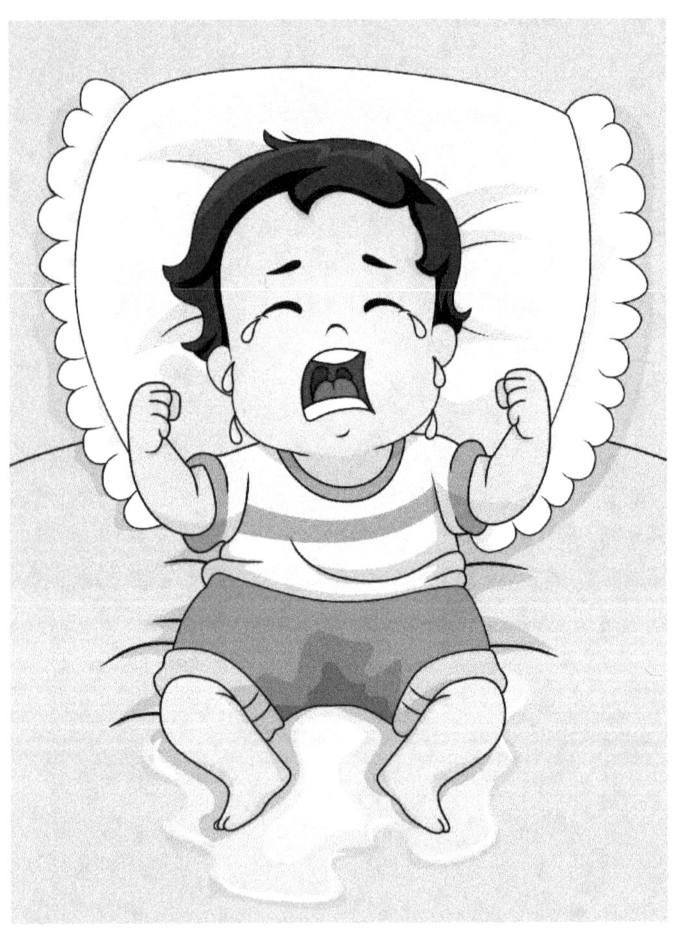

$\mathcal{I}$n this part, we'll examine the common medical complications that may affect the child's sleep or sleep training. There are lots of health issues that can cause sleep disorders when undetected, e.g. colic, allergies, teething, sleep apnea, etc. Under this section, we'll list the common medical complications that affect sleep, their causes and treatment. There are also some environmental conditions that may affect sleep in babies which will also be examined.

Medical Complications That Affect Sleep

In this section, we'll examine the medical complications that may affect your baby's sleep. If you notice your child has trouble sleeping all of a sudden, or if there is a sudden change in her sleep habits, a medical complication might be the cause. Below are the common medical complications that affect sleep:

1. Colic

Colic can be simply said to be a situation where a child suddenly starts to undergo long fussy periods without any obvious cause. It is not a disease but rather a series of surprising behaviors; for example, the child may suddenly begin to cry for more than three hours a day and for more than three days in a week. In other words, the baby cries a lot for long periods for what seems like no reason. According to research, colic usually starts when the baby is around two weeks old (for full-term babies) and may start later if the baby is premature. The baby's sex or feeding doesn't affect the occurrence but it usually resolves by the time the baby is 3 to 4 months old.

The symptoms include sudden loud cries, crying with clenched fists and flailing legs, crying for at least three hours at once, and the occurrence of these crying episodes for at least three days a week and three weeks in a row. The baby usually begins crying at the same time every day for no reason. He might have been well fed and might be in clean clothes and diapers but continues to cry for no reason. The baby may spit or pass gas during the episode. Colic greatly affects the baby's sleep as he continues to cry inconsolably during the day or at nighttime.

Colic has no known exact cause, although there have been a number of suggestions as to what may influence it. These include digestive issues such as gas buildup, gastroesophageal reflux disease (GERD), allergies or sensitivity, nervous system problems, unchecked injuries and infection. These are some of the theories developed to explain the factors behind colic. Meanwhile, there is still no exact reason for the condition.

Since there is no exact cause for colic, there is also no exact remedy. You may have to combine different approaches to make sure your baby calms down. However, the best thing is to visit a doctor who will then perform an examination to check for any underlying health issue. In managing the condition, it is important to try the methods one at a time, but with space between them so as not to overstimulate the baby. You may need to dim the lights and reduce noise, speak in soothing tones, or apply a little pressure to the baby's abdomen to help him relieve gas. You can swaddle and rock him until he calms down. A baby with colic will need extra effort and time to sleep at night so you should be prepared. It can be really frustrating to hear your baby cry for hours at a time so it is very important that you do not lose your cool. Remember, you should visit a doctor once you notice the symptoms of colic just to be safe.

2.   Teething

Teething is a normal part of the baby's growth and development, but the process is still largely uncomfortable for babies. Sleep problems usually occur during teething as the baby is too uncomfortable to fall asleep. Usually, babies start to teethe at around four to seven months of age, though teething at four months is quite rare. The first teeth usually start to appear at six months in most babies and come in gradually until the baby has the full set. Usually, the front incisors will appear first with the bottom front teeth or the top two. These will later be followed by the canines, and the eight molars usually appear between the age of one and three.

The common symptoms include: swollen or tender gums, crying, increased body temperature, gnawing on objects, drooling, and irritability. Diarrhea, vomiting, fever, and rashes are symptoms of other conditions and arc not normal signs of teething. If your baby develops these symptoms, you might need to visit a doctor. Your baby is very likely to get cranky at this time as teething is painful. She might be quick to cry during this period, so you'll need to spend more time soothing her rather than leaving her to self-soothe. You should also be prepared for lots of drooling, as teething stimulates saliva.

Though teething is a natural part of the baby's development, there are some things you can do to help ease the baby's discomfort. To start with, you can feel the baby's gums for bumps to check if the teeth are about to erupt. When you are sure that your baby is teething, you can take a clean, wet washcloth, place it in a plastic bag and refrigerate it for some minutes. You can then bring it out and allow the baby to gnaw on it. This will greatly help in relieving the pressure on his gums. This method can be applied before bedtime and nap time to make sure the baby gets enough uninterrupted sleep. Another method is to use a teething ring which can be placed in the refrigerator to cool before giving to the baby. This is a common and effective method used by many parents to relieve teething pain.

There are also some teething gels that can be applied on the gums to reduce the pressure temporarily. However, you should avoid teething gels that contain benzocaine, as it can cause dangerous side effects for babies under two. You can also consult your doctor to get some suitable pain meds for your baby.

3.   Nightmares and Bad Dreams During Naptime

Nightmares and night terrors are among the common sleep disturbances experienced by babies and toddlers, but they are quite different. Nightmares are typically bad or scary dreams that wake a child up from sleep. The child may wake up visibly scared or screaming as a result of a nightmare. If the baby is old enough to communicate, he or she will remember the dream and may want to tell you about it. Such a child might have trouble going back to sleep after experiencing a nightmare.

Nightmares typically occur during the second part of the night during REM (Rapid Eye Movement) sleep, usually close to morning. According to the National Sleep Foundation, about 25 percent of children between the ages of 5 and 12 experience frequent nightmares. Children usually begin to experience nightmares and night terrors at the age of 2, with most episodes occurring between the ages of 3 and 6.

Nightmares are usually influenced by daytime events, but they may also be caused by stress or separation anxiety. Nightmares and night terrors can also be triggered by sleep deprivation, inconsistent sleep schedule, or fever.

Night terrors usually happen during non-REM deep sleep, usually a few hours after your child goes to sleep. A night terror might last for up to 45 minutes and can occur many times in a night. The child might scream or panic while asleep. Even though his eyes may be open, he will be hard to console as they are still in deep sleep and oblivious to your presence. He won't remember them when he wakes up.

For nightmares, attend to the child as fast as possible if she has an episode. Hold the child and reassure her until she goes back to sleep. You might need to avoid scary stories before bedtime to prevent this. There has been some research on how temperature can influence nightmares; some studies suggest people are more likely to experience nightmares when sleeping in a cold room. The National Sleep Foundation recommends setting the temperature at 65F for restful sleep.

If your child experiences night terrors, the best thing to do is to wait it out while staying with him to prevent him from hurting himself. Usually, the child will go back to sleep without your intervention after a night terror.

4. Allergies and Food Intolerance

Allergies and food intolerance are among the health factors that can affect sleep in babies. Like adults, babies can experience several allergies and food intolerance. They can be allergic to objects, particles, and foods. These allergies are majorly classified under three categories: environmental allergies, food and medicine allergies, and seasonal allergies. Food and medicine allergies refer to allergic reactions which occur a while after the baby consumes a particular food he is allergic to.

Environmental allergies refer to things that can cause a reaction when the baby comes into contact with them such as dust, detergent, dander, etc. Seasonal allergies refer to allergic reactions that occur during specific parts of the year, especially allergic reactions to plants or trees that grow during a particular season.

Food allergies are the most common type of allergies seen in babies. The most common signs include itching, rashes or hives, wheezing and shortness of breath, face, tongue, or lip swelling, vomiting, diarrhea, and flushed skin. The common food items that may cause allergic reactions in babies include: peanuts, eggs, cow milk, tree nuts, fish, shellfish, soy, and wheat. Allergic reactions to these may range from mild to severe. Environmental allergies include allergic reactions to insect stings, dust, pollen, and mold.

According to the American Academy of Pediatrics, it is safe to introduce the food items mentioned above once the child is ready to take solid food. However, these foods should be introduced one at a time to be sure that they are safe for the baby. If you notice any food allergy symptoms in your baby, it is advisable to visit your pediatrician just to be safe. Some allergies may fade away with time while others may get progressively worse. For the first 6 months, it is recommended to breastfeed your baby to prevent a milk allergy.

The best way to prevent allergies is to eliminate contact with the allergen. If you are breastfeeding, some allergens might get to the baby through your breast milk, so it's important to check your diet also. If you notice your child has trouble sleeping or is irritable, you should check him for allergic reaction symptoms as they can be one of the factors that cause sleep problems.

5.   Sleep Apnea

Sleep apnea refers to a breathing disorder in which breathing stops partially or totally for a short period. Partial breathing reductions are called hypopneas while complete stops in breathing are called apneas. In children, the frequency of sleep apnea increases during REM sleep. The breathing problem usually happens as a result of an obstruction in the airway which may be caused by large tonsils and adenoids which obstruct the child's airway. The glands in the throat might also be infected and inflamed, thereby blocking the airway during sleep.

Typically, there are three infant sleep apneas: central, mixed, and obstructive apnea. Central apneas are a type of breathing problem in which the body reduces or stops the effort to breathe. This is usually as a result of a problem in the part of the brain controlling sleep, or a cardiac issue. Obstructive apneas are airway blockages caused by soft tissue collapse or inflammation during sleep. Mixed apneas are a combination of obstructive and central apneas. The obstructive apnea happens after the central apnea in this case. Central apneas are more common in full-term infants.

Sleep apneas can cause severe complications such as hypoxemia (low oxygen), irregular heartbeat and loss of consciousness. The symptoms of sleep apnea in infants include: mouth breathing, loud snoring, restlessness during sleep, and pausing of breathing. As for the treatment, you'll need to visit a doctor who will give a specific treatment based on the child's age, cause and severity of the condition. If the child has enlarged tonsils or adenoids, surgery is usually the best treatment. The child will undergo a tonsillectomy (removal of the tonsils) or adenoidectomy (removal of the adenoids). Sometimes, sleep apnea might be caused by obesity, though this is not common in children. If this is the case, you'll need to place the child on a weight loss plan. You should always check on your child periodically during sleep to see if he is breathing properly. If the child is experiencing a central apnea, you need to wake him up to resettle. Changing the sleeping position can also help to reduce the frequency of sleep apneas in toddlers.

6.   Restless Leg Syndrome

Restless leg syndrome refers to a sensory disorder which causes an unpleasant feeling and an irresistible urge to move the legs. This usually happens during bedtime but the child can experience the urge at other times as well, like after the legs have been stationary for a long time. The exact cause of restless leg syndrome isn't known yet, but it is often attributed to a low iron level, diabetes, or a neurological disorder. Some studies suggest restless leg syndrome is genetic and may be an inherited condition. It has also been suggested that it is a side effect of some drugs.

The symptoms of restless leg syndrome include an unpleasant sensation in the legs which includes itching, cramping, creeping, crawling, tingling, burning, and pain in general, leading to an almost irresistible urge to move the legs while sitting or lying down. The child may try to rub, turn, jiggle or stretch his legs to ease the uncomfortable feeling. The child will then need additional time to fall asleep as a result of these symptoms, and even after she falls asleep, she may have a hard time staying asleep because of the discomfort. Children with restless leg syndrome will also have trouble keeping the bedtime routines. They may get out of bed during bedtime to move their legs so as to ease the discomfort. This leads to a lot of bedtime behavior problems, especially if the child can't describe how she feels.

These bedtime problems may then lead to daytime sleepiness and behavioral problems as sleep deprivation causes irritability, moodiness, and inability to concentrate. Restless leg syndrome can, however, be managed through lifestyle changes and medication. To reduce the frequency in bed, the child should only go to bed once it's bedtime. Caffeinated products can also increase the frequency of restless leg syndrome, so they should be avoided. Cold compresses, heating pads, and massagers can be used on the legs to relieve the discomfort. You should also visit the doctor, who will prescribe the necessary micronutrients supplements such as iron supplements and folic acid.

7.   Sleep Problems in Premature Babies

By definition, a premature baby is one who is born at less than 37 weeks of gestation. The sleep schedules of preterm babies are quite different from that of full-term babies. Preterm babies typically sleep for a longer time than full-term infants. Though they are able to sleep longer than full-term infants, their sleep patterns take a longer time to develop and are largely inconsistent. They develop noticeable sleep patterns at a later time. According to a study on preterm infants, they are less able to show clear distress signals and are easily over-stimulated and stressed compared to full-term babies. They also exhibit markers of biobehavioral disorganization very frequently, i.e. they show a very limited range of interactional and attention skills compared to full-term infants. Another study suggested that preterm infants need more naps for proper growth and development.

Preterm infants also have a higher chance of being diagnosed with sleep apnea than full-term infants. Premature toddlers have a greater risk of developing sleep problems than healthy full-term infants, but they tend to learn to self-soothe easily. Preterm infants below the age of 21 months usually experience sleep problems like nocturnal movement, breathing problems, and restlessness. Though they need less help in falling asleep, they experience more sleep difficulties during the night. Preterm babies generally sleep more than full-term infants but with very low quality of sleep. They sleep for up to 22 hours per day but only sleep lightly.

Preterm babies will need a lot of help to stay comfortable. For example, a preterm child will need an incubator to help stay warm for some time after birth as they have little to no protective fat. They also need a ventilator in most cases to ensure the steady supply of oxygen and to prevent breathing problems such as apnea. A doctor is in the best position to determine the best methods to care for a preterm baby. A preterm baby will require more attention than a full-term baby, largely due to their fragility and developmental state. For example, a preterm child may not cry out loud enough for you to hear if there's a sleep disturbance, so there is the need for the parent to be very alert.

8.   Sleep Talking

Sleep talking, as the name implies, refers to the act of chattering or speaking during sleep. It is quite common in both infants and adults with different variations of length and audibility. Studies have shown that half of children between 3 and 10 years old talk while asleep. It either happens each night or at random occasions. Though sleep talking is generally harmless, it might be linked to some health conditions or sleep disorders in some cases. Sleep talking has been said to be genetic by researchers but can also be caused by stress and fatigue. It is also linked with nightmares, night terrors, and vivid dreams. Sleep talking usually starts in children between the ages of 2 and 3 and commonly occurs during deep sleep.

Sleep talking isn't usually a serious medical condition and most children will grow out of it within a short time. However, sleep talking can be reduced through healthy sleep habits. Since sleep talking is usually a sign of over-tiredness, it is important to make sure the child gets a quality nap each day and also keeps to a consistent bedtime routine.

9. Sleepwalking

Sleepwalking in infants, also known as pediatric sleepwalking or somnambulism, is a condition where a child wakes up from sleep and stands or walks without being aware. Though the child walks around, he isn't conscious and will not remember once he wakes up. Sleepwalking is more common in children between the ages of 4 and 8 and usually begins within an hour or two after the child goes to bed. In most kids, sleepwalking incidents usually last for around five to fifteen minutes. Though the condition is generally harmless, the child might get into dangerous situations if he sleepwalks while unattended. Waking a sleepwalking child up is generally not advised as it can be disorienting for them, and it is usually very difficult to wake sleepwalking children. Sleepwalking behaviors range from harmless to potentially harmful to inappropriate. In harmless sleepwalking, the child might just sit up in bed while he is not fully conscious. Potentially harmful sleepwalking involves the child walking around. Inappropriate sleepwalking episodes are when the child performs some "funny" actions while unconscious.

Sleepwalking is mostly caused by a number of factors, which include fatigue, sleep deprivation, bad sleeping habits, stress, illness, anxiety, reaction to some medications, and genetic factors. At times, sleepwalking may be a symptom of some other conditions like restless leg syndrome, sleep apnea, migraine, and bedwetting. During a sleepwalking episode, the child may sleep talk, sit up in bed, walk around the house, mumble during sleep, be unresponsive, perform inappropriate actions, or repeat some actions like sitting up, rubbing the eyes, or saying a word.

If there is no underlying condition causing sleepwalking in your child, then there is no need for treatment. The episodes will stop as the child gets older. However, there are some ways to reduce the frequency of sleepwalking. First, there is a method called scheduled awakening. It involves taking note of the usual time the sleepwalking episodes occur and waking the child up few minutes beforehand to reset his sleep cycle. There are some other preventive measures like keeping consistent sleep habits and avoiding caffeine and sugar before bed. The room can also be protected with safety barriers to prevent the child from harming himself.

10. Noisy Breathing in Babies

Noisy breathing is quite common in newborn babies as their respiratory system isn't fully developed yet. Newborns generally go through irregular breathing patterns which alternate between slow and fast rhythms and are accompanied by noises. This is because the respiratory pathways are still very narrow and get blocked easily. They also usually breathe through their tiny nostrils rather than from their mouths. Newborns take between 30 to 60 breaths per minute, which narrows down to around 25 to 40 breaths per minute by the time they are 6 months old. During sleep, babies might take rapid breaths and pause for some seconds, which might look strange to new parents. The child's breathing becomes more normal by the time they are six months.

Though some breathing noises are normal depending on the child's age, some other sounds might indicate an underlying medical condition. This is why you should take note of her normal breathing patterns to help determine if there's anything strange. A whistling noise usually signifies a blockage in the nostrils. You'll need to clear her nostrils by suctioning the mucus out, as newborns only breathe through their noses. It is also easy for their narrow nasal passages to get clogged, which will lead to a whistling noise. Fast, labored breathing might be a sign of pneumonia, and wheezing is a major sign of bronchitis or asthma.

In older babies, noisy breathing might be a sign of sleep apnea, asthma, bronchitis or some respiratory infections. In this case, you'll need to visit the doctor for diagnosis as the child might not be getting enough oxygen during sleep.

Environmental Factors That Affect Sleep

Having examined the medical factors that may affect sleep in children, you should also know about the environmental factors that may affect your baby's sleep. Sleep can be affected by hot and cold temperatures, trips, and potty training. We'll go through how all these affect sleep in children and what you should do.

1. Sleep During Summer and Winter (How Temperature Affects Sleep)

Sleep During Winter

During winter, babies sleep better and for periods as a result of the cool temperature. Naturally, the body temperature drops at night and the hormone melatonin is released during sleep. The baby's temperature is usually lowest at around 4 a.m. and the body starts preparing to wake up. Regardless, babies still need to be kept warm during winter. The baby should be dressed in enough clothes to keep them warm without a blanket as they can kick them off. The baby's face and head should be left bare to prevent the risk of suffocation. A safe infant sleeping bag can also be used.

Ironically, the most common risk babies face during winter according to studies is overheating. Most parents tend to dress their babies in overly thick clothes and blankets, which leads to overheating. Overheating puts babies at the risk of sudden infant death in severe cases. It can also cause irritability, dehydration, and discomfort in babies. You should adjust the baby's clothes and blankets according to his body temperature. You can do this by placing your hand on the child's abdomen. If he feels too warm, reduce the layer of clothing, and vice versa. The temperature shouldn't be too hot or cold. The ideal temperature for babies is between 68 F to71 F. It can be adjusted based on your baby's body temperature.

Sleep During Summer

Babies are also at the risk of overheating during summer due to the higher temps, and due to the fact that they cannot regulate their body temperature like adults can. Hot temperatures put babies at the risk of SIDS and can reduce the quality of sleep. The body temperature naturally goes down at night during sleep, which improves the quality of sleep. However, during summer, the increased temperature can cause a spike in the baby's body temperature, causing sleep problems. Most pediatricians recommend using an air conditioner during the day and a fan at night to keep the baby cool. The increased period of daylight can also affect the baby's natural sleep cycles, so it's important to get blackout curtains to help support the baby's circadian rhythm.

2. Trips

Sleep during trips can be a different ballgame for babies due to the change in environment and the absence of the usual sleep training materials. Regression can also happen during trips and you should prepare for that. When traveling to a new location, the baby might have a hard time falling asleep or sleeping for long, as the body naturally tries to stay alert when in a new environment. Regardless, you should try as much as possible to mimic the usual sleep training routines you practice at home. Before going on car trips, make sure the baby is well rested before moving out of the house, since an overtired or irritable baby will not be calm during a trip.

3. Lack of Naptime

A child who doesn't get a proper nap during the day will have some trouble sleeping at night. On average, babies need more than 10 hours of sleep per day with between one to three or four naps depending on the age. Lack of naptime will lead to an overtired and irritable baby who will have trouble sleeping at night. Babies who experience sleep deprivation due to insufficient naptime will have trouble feeding properly. Such babies will wake up at random times during the night to feed again. Babies and toddlers need a sufficient amount of daytime naps in order to keep proper nighttime sleeping habits.

The child should have a daytime sleep routine which is in line with his natural sleep cycle. Naps are also very important in maintaining alertness and concentration in children.

4. Oversleeping

Oversleeping is a situation when a child sleeps for more than the recommended number of hours per day. For example, newborns should sleep for 14 to 17 hours per day according to the National Sleep Foundation, but some newborns may sleep for up to 19 hours per day due to some factors. Oversleeping can happen as a result of a disruption in the normal sleep routine or if the child has a health issue. Oversleeping also happens during a growth spurt or a developmental leap as the body releases the growth hormone during sleep. Immunization and respiratory infections also cause children to sleep for long periods. Oversleeping might be a way for the child to compensate for low quality sleep. Oversleeping under normal conditions isn't considered harmful, but you have to make sure the child gets enough food before he goes back to sleep.

In some cases, oversleeping can be a result of jaundice or malnutrition. The baby might become lethargic and too tired to stay awake and will then sleep more than usual. Preterm babies also sleep longer than full-term babies. For newborns, you can keep a sleep log and a feeding log to track the baby's sleep and feeding schedules. You might need to wake the baby up to eat sometimes. If the baby shows signs of health issues, then it's advisable to visit a doctor.

5. Bedwetting

Bedwetting in babies and toddlers is not considered a serious problem, especially in babies. The bladder is not large enough to hold urine overnight. Meanwhile, the feeling of being wet is quite uncomfortable for babies and they may wake up from sleep moments after peeing themselves. You'll need to get absorbent underpants which could be disposable or reusable plus sleeping bag liners. These would help in reducing the wet sensation the baby feels after bedwetting. If the child is older, you can cut down on the food and drink he takes before bed, drinks especially. Toddlers can be woken up periodically and encouraged to ease their bladder. For much younger children, especially newborns, there is nothing much to do except to get absorbent underwear or diapers which will lessen the wet feeling.

You might not need to change the child's underwear or diaper during the night except if he's too wet or if you can do it gently without waking him up.

All Sorts Of Weaning

In this chapter, we'll go through the different sorts of weaning, how it affects the child, and how to do it.

1. Night Weaning

Night weaning refers to reducing the amount of nighttime feedings until they stop completely. Night weaning helps the baby sleep longer since he will no longer need to feed at night. Though it varies, most babies are usually ready for night weaning between the ages of four and six months. At this stage, they can store enough calories to sustain them for five to six hours during the night without waking up to feed. In some cases, babies younger than four months can sleep through the night without waking up to feed, while some babies older than 4 months still wake up to feed. It all depends on the baby and the parent. The baby might need night feedings during an illness, teething, or a growth spurt. Even sleep-trained children might need night feedings during these periods.

The weaning process should be done gradually to make it easy for the child. The night feedings should be reduced bit by bit until the child is ready to sleep through the night. Sometimes it becomes a habit for the baby to wake up to feed during the night, so it'll take some time to correct this. Some pediatricians have suggested that night feedings may cause some sleep problems. Pediatrician Dr. Richard Ferber says waking up a baby to feed several times during the night might lead to a very wet diaper which will cause the child to wake up more. This leads to a cycle of sleeping, feeding, and waking.

However, some pediatricians suggest night feedings may help to strengthen the bond between parents and children and that parents shouldn't rush through night weaning. One way to make the transition from night feeding to night weaning is to make sure the child has enough to eat through the day. Make sure you have a quiet feeding session with the baby during daytime to make sure he gets enough food. You might need to offer him extra feedings to ensure he goes to bed with a full stomach. However, feeding shouldn't be the last bedtime activity, to prevent it from becoming a habit. After this, gradually eliminate night feedings bit by bit until the child can sleep through the night without needing to feed.

2. Weaning Off the Pacifier

Though the pacifier is great for soothing babies, there will be a time when the baby will get too old for it and you'll have to wean him off it. This might not be easy, especially if the child has gotten used to it, but there are some methods you can apply to make it easier. The child shouldn't be weaned off the pacifier until he is at least a year old. According to the American Academy of Pediatrics, pacifiers help to reduce the risk of sudden infant death syndrome when used at naptime and at bedtime during a child's first year. The child may also need the pacifier when going through a major life change as it helps him self-soothe during these periods. However, your child may need to let go of the pacifier if he suffers from frequent ear infections as continued usage can lead to a buildup of fluid in the middle ear. The child may also need to stop using the pacifier immediately if he has teeth and mouth problems as a result of frequent usage, or if he has speech and language problems.

There are many ways to go about weaning children off the pacifier. One is the cold turkey method. In this method, you simply take away the pacifier and stop the child from using it henceforth. This method isn't suitable for everyone as there may be a lot of crying and temper tantrums from the child, who might wake up at night and cry for the pacifier. If you are prepared for this, then you can adopt the method. Before and after taking the pacifier away, it is still advisable to explain to the child what you are about to do. Regardless, you have to keep to your word once you take the pacifier away for the method to be effective.

Another method is the phase-it-out method. In this method you set gradual limits on when and where the pacifier will be used. This slow and gentle weaning process is easier for the child and she will stop using it eventually. Another method is to exchange the pacifier for a toy, or whatever the child wants and you are comfortable with. After you take the pacifier, replace it with the reward. There is a common method in which you put a bitter or unpleasant but safe substance on the pacifier. With a few attempts, the child will learn to stay away from the pacifier on her own.

3. Weaning Off Being Rocked to Sleep

Babies who can't go to sleep independently will need some assistance like swaddling or rocking to sleep. However, a time will come when you'll need to stop this. The process is not an overnight one; it might take some time for the baby to fully adjust. As your baby gets bigger, rocking might become tiresome for you and also take longer time for the baby to go to sleep. Rocking becomes a habit easily for babies, and with time, your baby will expect to be rocked to sleep each time he wakes up during the night. Once the baby is over four months, it is advisable to reduce your reliance on rocking to get him to sleep. At this stage, he starts to develop self-soothing. However, in babies over five months old, rocking to sleep is actually one of the reasons they stay awake in the night. Babies this age wake between sleep cycles and might need to soothe themselves before going back to sleep. However, if the baby is used to being rocked to sleep, he will not go back to sleep until you rock him.

Since weaning the baby from being rocked to sleep is a gradual process, there are some steps you need to take in the right order. First, it is advisable to start with rocking the baby until she becomes drowsy before placing her in the crib. As opposed to rocking her until she falls totally asleep, you can start with rocking her until she becomes sleepy, then placing her in the crib. If the baby fusses, you can touch her or make a gentle rubbing motion to calm her down. The next step is to only hold the baby until she becomes drowsy. You can rock for a bit to calm her down, but after that, hold the baby still until she becomes drowsy, after which you can place her in the crib to fall asleep totally. Also, when the baby wakes up during the night, you can lift her from the crib and hold her without rocking, then once she becomes drowsy, place her in the crib again. You can gradually move from lifting the child out of the crib to holding her in the crib.

Another method practiced by some parents is to wake him from sleep and let him fall asleep on his own without rocking. This encourages the child to self-soothe, and with time, there will no longer be the need to rock the child to sleep. Regardless of the method you prefer, you need consistency to get the desired results. You should use the same method during daytime and nighttime.

4. Weaning Off Swaddling

Though there is no specific age for a child to stop being swaddled, most children are usually ready to stop by the time they are four months old. Though swaddling, when done correctly, can help to soothe your baby, it also comes with some risks if done incorrectly. Some studies also suggest swaddling may pose some health risks, such as affected arousal thresholds and lower respiratory tract infection, though these have not been fully confirmed. By the time the baby is four months old, he will have lost what is known as the Moro reflex, so there might not be the need for you to swaddle him any longer. Also, if the baby is old enough to roll over, then you'll need to stop swaddling him.

Before you start to wean the baby off swaddling, you need to determine an alternative you can employ in place of the method. The most usual alternative is the sleeping bag. This helps to keep the baby warm through the night and reduces the risk of suffocation from loose sheets or blankets. This method involves three steps. The first step is to swaddle the child over a sleeping bag to get him used to it. After that, wrap the baby with his arms out but make sure the blankets aren't loose. The last step is to place the child in the sleeping bag without swaddling him. Once the child can sleep comfortably without being swaddled, then the process is complete.

5. Weaning Off Sleep Schedule Management

You may get tired of keeping track of the child's sleeping schedule or keeping a sleep log and you'll long for the time the child will learn to sleep independently. This all starts from the sleep training and the sleep schedule you create for your child. Any sleep schedule you create must fall in line with the child's natural sleep patterns. This, along with a consistent and comfortable bedtime routine, will become a habit for the child and as he grows older, he'll learn to go to bed himself without you needing to manage his sleep schedule. One important thing you must note is that sleep cycles change as the child grows older. For example, the number of naps the child needs to take reduces as he grows older, as does the duration. The key is to create a sleep schedule which is age appropriate and comfortable for the child. According to the National Sleep Foundation, babies between 0-2 months should get around 10 to 18 hours of sleep per day. For children around 3 to 12 months, 9.5 to 14 hours of sleep is enough, children around 1-3 years old should get between 12 to 14 hours of sleep each day, and 11-13 hours of sleep is adequate for children around 3 to 5 years old.

Create a consistent bedtime routine and help the child keep to it. As the child grows older, he'll become used to it and you will no longer need to manage his sleep schedule. However, you may still need to check periodically to make sure he gets the recommended amount of sleep.

PART FIVE

***

FAQ

A Better Place for Your Baby's Sleep

Where the baby sleeps is largely dependent on her age. Older babies may no longer need to sleep in a crib. According to the American Academy of Pediatrics, a baby should sleep in either a bassinet, a cradle, or crib that is not too far from the parent for the first six months. The baby should always be positioned to sleep on their back to reduce the risk of sudden infant death syndrome (SIDS). The crib mattress should be firmly fitted and should be covered with a firm sheet. Soft objects like pillows, loose bedding, or other blankets should not be kept in the crib or bassinet to reduce the risk of suffocation. Toys also should not be kept in the crib.

The baby shouldn't sleep on the same bed with you to prevent accidental suffocation, according to the American Academy of Pediatrics. The best way to stay close to your baby for the first six months is to share a room but not a bed with the baby. This way, you'll be able to attend to him quickly and also monitor him properly. The sleeping area (bassinet, crib, or cradle) should have a wide base and should not be easy to knock down. The sides should be around 15 inches tall and the crib must be properly assembled. Most parents move their babies into another room after 6 months but it is okay to wait longer, provided the room is safe for the baby.

There are some unsafe places for the child to sleep in the home. The first is the living room furniture. Studies have shown that babies who sleep on living room furniture have up to 67 times the risk of sudden infant death syndrome. The same goes for babies who sleep on recliners, armchairs, cushions, or beanbag chairs. Apart from living room furniture, car seats are also among the most dangerous places for your baby to sleep, since the baby can roll over while dozing upright and might face breathing difficulties.

Why Is It Important to Shade the Room During Sleep?

You've probably read many childcare articles that encourage parents to shade the child's room. You may wonder if it actually is important and how it affects the child's sleep. It actually has many advantages. First, babies need some darkness to sleep comfortably. Shading the room causes the pineal gland to release the hormone melatonin, which helps the body relax until they fall asleep. Bright lights can affect the baby's circadian rhythm as it makes it harder for them to fall asleep. One efficient way to get your baby to sleep is to use blackout curtains which will filter out the natural lights, especially during daytime. There are some blackout drapes specially designed to filter out outside noise. This type of curtain performs a double function: it darkens the room and also filters noise.

Thermal curtains help to prevent sunlight from getting into the room and heating it up. These are very useful during the summer when the temperature is particularly high. Thermal curtains are also very useful during the winter as they can keep the heat in the room from getting out while blocking the cold air outside. When using blackout curtains during the day, the room shouldn't be totally dark so as not to confuse the baby, as daytime might look like nighttime, which isn't good for the child's sleep cycle. The room should be dimly lit and free from noise instead.

Noise and Music: Harm or Benefit?

Many parents use white noise to help their child sleep better at night, and there has been a lot of debate on the benefits and disadvantages of its long-term use. Before talking about the cons, let's examine how white noise affects the baby. While in the womb, babies experience some form of a low frequency noise from the beating heart, the blood flowing through the body, the flow of air into the lungs, exhaling, etc. This according to researchers can be as loud as 80 decibels. After the baby is born, he finds himself in an environment filled with strange noises from multiple sources, and this can be disconcerting. Total silence as well as loud noises can also affect the baby's sleep negatively, as the baby is used to the low frequency sounds from the womb. In research conducted by the National Institute of Health in which 20 babies were studied, it was discovered that 80% of the infants fell asleep within five minutes under white noise, while the rest fell asleep spontaneously.

If you live in a crowded city, the loud noises will surely affect your baby's sleep in one way or the other. The sounds from a white noise machine drown out other surrounding noise, which creates a very comfortable environment similar to that of the womb for the baby. There are even some white noise machines made specifically for infants with lullabies, heartbeat sounds to mimic the parent's, and other soothing sounds. White noise has been found to help babies fall asleep easily and to stay asleep for longer periods. From a study published in the Archives of Diseases in Childhood, it was determined that white noise can encourage sleep in children. From a careful observation of the sleep habits of forty newborns under white noise, it was seen that up to 80 percent of children fall asleep within five minutes under white noise.

White noise helps to drown out disturbing sounds that may affect the baby's sleep, especially during the end of a sleep cycle, when the baby is more likely to wake. White noise machines also help to drown out household noises coming from appliances, other members of the house, and siblings. This is particularly useful for households where there are many children who sleep at different times. Also, a completely silent environment can cause babies to feel isolated or scared. White noise machines prevent this by creating a soothing background noise to keep the baby comfortable.

Despite its advantages, white noise and music have some drawbacks too. First, in a study conducted on white noise use in different households, it was determined that most white noise machines exceed the recommended 50-decibel limit for babies. This can lead to hearing loss and may even affect the baby's sleep negatively. Also, some babies can become "addicted" to white noise and cannot fall asleep easily without it. In a situation where white noise or music isn't available, the child can experience sleep deprivation. Lastly, not all babies adapt to white noise. Some babies find it hard to sleep with white noise and continued usage will affect the baby's sleep patterns. Regardless, the benefits of white noise or soothing music can outweigh the drawbacks when used correctly.

Why Massage Is Important for a Child

Massage or infant massage is among the many methods of calming or relaxing a child before bed. The importance of a gentle massage before bedtime is greatly underestimated by many parents. According to research, gentle massages can be a way to help a baby maintain their circadian rhythm. A proper circadian rhythm involves more hours of nighttime sleep and sufficient daytime activity. A number of physical and mental changes like temperature, sleep, and daytime activity are influenced by the circadian rhythm. It even influences the child's appetite. When the body prepares for sleep once daytime fades, the hormone melatonin is released to help the baby calm down and make him fall asleep easily. This hormone is constantly released throughout the night and increases with the amount of sleep the baby gets. A gentle massage can help increase the levels of this hormone.

A massage can help relieve stress and tension in children and adults. It helps to relax and calm the baby when it's time for bed. This is particularly helpful for very active babies or overtired babies. Massage has also been found to relieve and calm babies suffering from colic. A massage can also be a way to bond with your child. That gentle touch can help promote a healthy emotional connection between you and your baby. Some studies have also shown some other benefits of massaging your baby such as healthy weight gain, improved immune function, and a healthy development. This is because sleep affects all the things mentioned and a massage helps the baby get quality sleep. Massaged infants fall asleep faster and also sleep for longer than infants who are not.

Massages help to lower the levels of the stress hormone also known as cortisol. Since the skin is filled with more than 5 million sensory receptors, the contact from a massage helps to calm the baby down and also increases the melatonin levels.

Bath Time Routine

Like massages, bathing can help babies sleep better when incorporated into the bedtime routine. Once warm baths have been made part of the baby's bedtime routine, it should not be skipped as it can affect the child's sleep negatively. However, a warm bath may not work for all babies, as it can achieve the opposite of what the parent desires; bedtime baths can keep some babies awake and alert. However, according to Dr. Jodi Mindell, a sleep medicine specialist and pediatric psychologist, warm baths followed by a gentle massage can help the baby get quality sleep as the baby will spend 25 percent less time crying after a warm bath. Dr. William Sears, a child care specialist and author, advises that once you make bath time a part of the bedtime routine and it works for your baby, you should stick with it.

A small plastic bath can be used. The baby must never be left alone during bath time, no matter how short the time will be. Warm baths should be one of the last bedtime activities for your baby. As many childcare experts have suggested, feeding shouldn't be the last bedtime activity. A warm bath followed by a lullaby or story can help get the child to sleep easily. The water must be around body temperature and you can use a thermometer or dip your hand in to check. After the bath, massage the child with baby lotion and dress him up for bedtime.

Types of Baby Cries and Why It Is Important to Listen

There are many reasons babies cry and this is reflected in the way they cry. Since babies cannot communicate verbally, the only medium of communication for them is crying. If you observe your baby carefully, you might be able to pinpoint what is wrong just from the way he cries. The following are the six ways to understand a baby's cries:

1. Rhythmic Crying

Rhythmic crying involves a low pitched and repetitive cry which usually signals that the baby is hungry. For most babies, the cry usually sounds like a low pitched "nehh." This is usually accompanied by other signs such as reaching for the breast, putting fingers in the mouth, and sucking motions. The peculiar sound comes from placing the tongue to the roof of the mouth and trying to suck. When your baby cries in this manner, the best thing to do is to attend to him immediately. The longer you wait, the more he will cry.

2. High-Pitched Shrieks

This type of cry is unforgettable for most parents as they immediately know that something is wrong. The cries are loud, ear piercing, and usually short depending on the cause of the pain, for example, during vaccine shots or gas pain.

Once you hear this type of cry, move to the baby as fast as possible and check for the source of the pain.

3.   The Whiny, Nasal Cry

This type of cry usually increases in intensity and is a sign that the baby is tired of whatever he's doing or is uncomfortable. This is usually accompanied by yawns and eye rubs. This occurs mostly when the baby needs to take a nap.

4.   The Fussy Cry

Sometimes babies cry because they are bored. You can notice this when the baby has been in a position or performing an activity for awhile. They only need to be taken away from the noise, movement or whatever is stressing them out.

5.   Colic

Colic is accompanied by loud and intense cries that go on for more than three hours. This usually occurs in the late afternoon or evening and starts before the baby is three months old. This type is the most frustrating for parents as it can go on for hours without a specific reason. To soothe the baby, you can gently rock or swaddle him. Colic usually ends by the time the baby is three to four months old.

6.   Whimpers

Nasal-sounding soft whimpers can be a sign that the baby is sick. This type of cry is lower pitched than the pain cry and is usually weak, due to the fact that the baby is too weak to cry loudly. If you notice this, check for other symptoms like fever, diarrhea, vomiting, or rashes. If so, you'll need to contact a doctor for diagnosis and treatment.

When should the child move to an adult bed?

Most babies are ready to move from a crib to a bed at around 18 months to 3 years of age. Though there is no specific time for the child to move to a bed, there are some signs that the child might be ready for the transition. First, if the child has overgrown the crib or there's a newborn baby in the house who might need it, then you may move the child into an adult bed. If the child has started trying to climb out of the crib or is undergoing potty training, then a bed might be easier. To lower the risk of accidents, it is advisable to switch to a bed once you notice your child has started trying to climb out. Before switching to a bed, make sure the room and the whole house is childproof. It is easy for the child to move around on a bed than in a crib. Remove potentially dangerous objects from the room and make sure the child doesn't have the chance to climb drawers and bookshelves. You should also prepare yourself for tantrums as the child may prefer his crib.

If you prefer to use a toddler bed, make sure it is low to the ground to reduce the risk of injuries from your child falling out. There are portable bed rails you can install which will prevent this. For adult beds, there should be no space between the mattress and the rail. You can put soft materials around the bed in case the child does fall out. As most experts recommend, the bed should be free from toys, especially for children under 2 years. To make the transition easier for your child, make sure the bed is positioned in the same way as the crib and the child uses the same blanket.

Why shouldn't the child be left to scream for more than 20 minutes?

When using sleep training methods like the cry-it-out method, you may decide to leave the child to cry it out for some time before attending to him. While this isn't bad, there are some limits you should set. The first is the child shouldn't be allowed to scream for more than 20 minutes before attending to him. Also, you might need to rush to the child earlier than usual if you notice a high-pitched cry, which may signal that the child is in pain. Though many studies have confirmed that leaving the child to cry for some time can help him develop self-soothing quickly, leaving a child to cry can cause problems when done for long periods.

According to a study published by childcare expert Penelope Leach, babies who are consistently left to cry for long periods of time are at more risk of suffering brain damage which might lead to learning difficulties and some other developmental difficulties. According to her, sometimes the baby might stop crying not because he has learned to soothe himself, but because he is simply too tired to cry. This prolonged stress leads to increased levels of the stress hormone cortisol in the body and very high levels of the hormone can cause brain damage. Another child care specialist, Dr. Sunderland, advises against prolonged crying in children. In her words:

The infant brain is so vulnerable to stress. After birth, it's not yet finished! In the first year of life, cells are still moving to where they need to be. This is a process known as migration, and it's hugely influenced by uncomforted stress. Then in the first year of life, there are adverse stress-related changes to the gene expression of key emotion chemical systems. They are responsible for the emotional well-being and the ability to be calm and handle stress well in later life.

According to studies, prolonged crying can lead to elevated blood pressure, irregular heartbeat, sleep problems, and increase in body temperature. Also, leaving your baby to cry for more than 20 minutes can lead to you missing some urgent issues you might need to attend to.

I can't stand my baby crying. What do I do?

This is the exact opposite of what we examined above. Many new mothers experience this and it's perfectly normal. Many parents simply can't stand their baby crying. Leaving him to cry for more than 30 seconds is terrifying to them, making them rush to attend to him as fast as possible. If you experience this, it is quite normal and very common. It must, however, be balanced to save yourself some stress and to help the baby learn how to self-soothe. According to some studies, the hormone oxytocin is released in large amounts during pregnancy and labor and it changes the way mothers process the sound of crying babies. It also helps them distinguish the sound easily from other sounds, allowing a mother to easily tell when a baby is crying even though he may be in another room.

This is why mothers develop a rapid reaction to a baby's cries. However, you need to balance this as attending to your baby immediately can cause separation anxiety in some cases. The baby can have a hard time learning to self-soothe if he is used to you coming immediately every time he cries. To manage this, you can set a timer which you keep strictly to. When the baby starts crying or fussing, time yourself to wait for two minutes or some other convenient amount of time before attending to him. You have to be consistent with this if you want your child to learn how to self-soothe.

My child isn't happy in the morning. Does he remember what happened at night?

Depending on the age of the baby, he may remember a long night or may not. Experts suggest babies can remember familiar faces and voices starting from the first two months. Babies who are being breastfed can recognize the mother's smell after just a week. While this is an indication of memory, it is still quite different from remembering specific events. **The baby might not start remembering** specific events until he is **around 14 to 18 months old**. Most times, a child being moody doesn't mean he remembers what happened after a bad night, it can simply be a sign of tiredness or sleep deprivation. Even if it looks like the child remembers, he's sure to forget within a short period of time. You should, however, make sure the child gets enough daytime sleep and you should also make an effort to ensure he sleeps comfortably each night.

Why is good sleep so difficult?

This is a question on the lips of many frustrated parents: "Why is a good night's sleep so difficult?" Good sleep shouldn't be difficult unless the baby suffers from colic or other illnesses that may make sleeping through the night a chore. All of the bedtime tips and methods you may have read online may not work if you don't modify them to suit your baby's temperament and sleep habits. In most cases, neither the parent nor the baby is at fault for the bedtime problems; the parent might have tried many different methods, all to no avail. The first thing you should do if your baby experiences regular bedtime problems is to check if she has any health issues as they can cause a lot of sleep problems and make sleep training difficult. You may also need to visit a pediatrician for diagnosis. If the pediatrician rules out any health issues, then you can be sure that it's just a matter of time, patience, and careful observation until the child begins to sleep comfortably.

The next thing to do is to **carefully observe the child.** Even if he experiences sleep problems, there will surely be times when he sleeps through the night comfortably. Pay attention to those times and look for what is missing in the other periods. Sometimes, the sleep training methods you adopted may not be suited to your baby's temperament, especially if the baby is a signaler. You just need to be patient and open to trying different bedtime routines until you find what works for your baby. You must avoid getting frustrated as it only makes it more difficult. With time and patience, the sleep problems will go away.

There are some helpful tips that can be useful in getting your baby to sleep comfortably. The first is to **avoid stimulation** and engaging activities close to bedtime. A warm bath or massage can help **relax** the baby and put him **in the mood to sleep.** It's easier for a calm and relaxed baby to go to sleep than an excited one. Also, you should keep a stable bedtime routine which should include relaxing activities like reading books. Sometimes, trying out too many methods and bedtime routines within a short period of time can be confusing for the baby. You should be consistent with a method until you are sure if it works or not.

I can't determine my child's temperament. What do I do?

There may be times when parents find it hard to pinpoint their child's temperament, thereby leading to difficulties in choosing the right sleep training method and bedtime routine for their baby. There are basically two ways to go about this. The first is to pay more attention to your child. In previous parts of the book, we have examined the different types of temperaments children possess. By carefully studying your baby and cross-checking the explained temperaments, you'll be able to determine your child's temperament in no time. If it still seems impossible, you may just need to wait for some time for the child to develop noticeable characteristics. There are also online tests you can take that will make it easier for you to determine your child's temperament. There are specialized and clear questions that make the process very easy.

Another method is to visit a childcare specialist who will help determine your child's temperament upon careful observation. The main factors that are important in determining a child's temperament include level of activity, approach and withdrawal, adaptability, mood, attention span, sensory threshold, self-soothing, etc. You should know that your child is either a signaler or a self-soother. As for the general temperaments in children, there are three types: the easygoing or laid-back child, the slow to warm up child, and the difficult or spirited (very active) child. Your child will fall under one of these three categories.

My child is very naughty; he doesn't follow any training.

There have been comments from frustrated parents about their child's unwillingness to follow any sleep training or bedtime routine. This is mostly common in children with dominant personalities or spirited children. While the child's temperament largely matters during sleep training, the approach also matters. It may also be due to other issues and not just the child being naughty. First, the child may just not be ready for sleep training. Children develop at different rates and are very unique, and you may think your baby is ready for sleep training when he is not. **Forcing sleep training on such a child will lead to a lot of problems**. In some situations, the child may actually be ready for sleep training but will only need a longer period to learn how to self-soothe.

Contrary to what some people believe, sleeping is very developmental and has a lot to do with how well a baby can regulate its melatonin production. The baby will need some help with this, though, and this is where sleep training comes in. Some babies might not be ready yet and are not stubborn, despite what their parents think. Also, the approach and bedtime routine clearly matter. If your approach isn't suited to your baby's temperament, there will be lots of problems with sleep training. There may also be some other issues you are not noticing. The sleep schedule might not be in line with his natural sleep cycle, the baby might be hungry during the training periods, or there are too many sleep training methods being used. Bedtime routines also have a large role to play in sleep training, especially for toddlers. The bedtime routine should be fun and relaxing for the baby and not something you have to force your baby to do. Regardless, you should also be consistent with the routines and methods you choose to adopt for your baby, provided they are suitable for him.

Why are there so many sleep training methods? Do you have to try everything?

It's easy to get confused by the many sleep training methods out there. You may be wondering if you need to try each of them before your child eventually learns to sleep through the night comfortably. However, the different sleep training methods were created for other reasons; you do not need to try them all. It all boils down to what the child is comfortable with. The reason why there are many ways to calm a child is because of the individual differences or temperaments in children. Each child is unique and what calms one child may not calm another. Even among siblings, you may need to adopt different training and soothing methods. Once you find a method that works well for your baby, it's advisable to stick with it.

Trying too many methods at once can actually prolong sleep training, as the child will need more time to adjust in between the sleep training methods. The best thing is to choose a method that matches your baby's personality and temperament. If the method doesn't seem to work, wait a bit before you try another method. The new method should be introduced gradually to make the change easy for the baby. Most times, the baby may just need a little more time to learn how to self-soothe. Regardless of which method you choose, it must be safe and comfortable for the baby.

My baby wants to sleep with us. What should I do?

This is a common question many parents ask: what do they do when the baby refuses to sleep alone or wants to sleep in their bed? Here's what child experts have to say. According to the American Academy of Pediatrics, bed sharing shouldn't be practiced due to the risk of accidental injury or suffocation. However, it is recommended that infants share their parents' bedroom at least for the first six months to a year. The baby should sleep on a different surface like a crib or bassinet and never on furniture. If you choose to sleep in the same bed as your child, she must be at least a year old, though it can still be risky. However, if you choose to co-share, the mattress must be very large, flat, and firm, with no space between it and the wall. Pillows and blankets should be removed and you might need to demarcate the sleeping area to prevent the child from rolling under you.

When you are ready to move the child to another room, you need to make the transition as easy as possible. Spend time together in the new room. It can be used for feedings, naps, or playtime. The child will get used to the room during this period, which will make the move more comfortable. If your child is still less than a year old, then it might be better to let him stay in the same room as you.

A Crib in the Parents' Bedroom After Six Months

After six months, the child may be ready to move into their own room. Studies have shown that babies who sleep in their own room after six months sleep more independently than babies who stay in the same room as their parent. Regardless, it is still safe for the baby to sleep in a parent's room for the first six months to around a year. There are some peculiar outcomes you may experience if you keep the child's crib in your bedroom after 6 months. First, the child may want to sleep close to you, i.e. in the same bed, which isn't recommended. If you want to keep a child in the same room as you after six months, then you have to make sure the room is safe for the baby. You also mustn't give in to the temptation of sleeping in the same bed as your baby.

Also, older children might attempt to climb out of the crib. Such children may need a toddler bed but not an adult one. In that case, the child will need to stay in another room for safety purposes. There is another way out of this, though: you can get a larger crib for the child if you are comfortable with it.

My baby doesn't stick to the feeding schedule and the same amounts. Is this a problem?

This is another common problem faced especially by parents who choose scheduled feeding over on-demand feeding. The child may refuse to eat or may eat very little during the scheduled feeding periods. To know if this is a problem or not, you have to track the child's overall daily intake. If the baby gets enough food each day while feeding at other periods not on the schedule, then it's not a problem.

However, if the baby does not get enough food, is losing weight, or is looking malnourished, then you might need to make some changes to the feeding schedule. A rigid feeding schedule can cause feeding problems. Most childcare experts recommend flexible schedules or even on-demand feeding. For babies under three months, on-demand feeding is needed. This is because their sleep and wake cycles are still irregular and they will need to feed every few hours.

After three months, flexible feeding schedules are more comfortable for parents, especially working parents. To make sure it stays convenient for both you and the baby, make sure the feeding schedule is in line with the child's natural feeding patterns. This will help make sure the child eats enough food at the expected period. Feed the baby in a quiet room so that he does not get distracted. If the child is feeling sleepy before the scheduled time, it's okay to feed him before then. However, it is important to note that there are periods when the feeding schedule might not be useful. The child's feeding schedule might change during growth spurts, illnesses, and some developmental changes. Remember, the key goal is to make sure your child gets enough calories to sustain him during the day and through the night.

I do not want to wake the child day or night. What should I do ?

If you prefer not to wake the child to feed during the day and at night, then scheduled feeding might not be suitable, especially if the baby still needs to feed during the night. Also, the wake and sleep training method might not be suitable. In this case, you should be prepared to attend to the child anytime he wakes up to feed. On-demand feeding is okay as long as the child gets enough. You can also go along with it as long as you have enough time to attend to the baby. If you do not want to wake the child at any time during the day and you prefer feeding on demand, there are some advantages that come with that. First, feeding on demand ensures the baby gets enough to eat. It also allows for more bonding time between you and the baby and ensures that the baby sleeps uninterrupted for as long as he is full.

There are some drawbacks to choosing not to wake your child. The first is that night feedings will go on for longer periods. The child may also take longer to learn to self-soothe, as he might associate feeding with bedtime. There will be times where you'll be left with no choice but to wake the baby. For example, if the baby's diaper is full, you need to change it, as it is not advisable to leave a baby in their excrement or urine for long. The baby might wake up during the process of changing the diaper. While on-demand feeding is very comfortable for the baby, it might be inconvenient for you in the long run.

Sleep and new siblings, how do I cope?

The arrival of new siblings can affect your child's sleep. She can also undergo some behavioral changes during this period, which is why it is very important to learn how to manage this situation to prevent problems. There are some helpful tips you should take note of to help your child adjust during the arrival of a new sibling. Most times, bringing in a new sibling causes some setbacks with the older sibling's sleep training. The first thing to do is to constantly remind the child that they are getting a brother/sister soon, to prepare them for the addition. During this period and after, you should provide your child with enough attention to prevent him from feeling neglected once the new child arrives. Sometimes, bedtime problems may occur when a new sibling arrives because the older sibling is feeling displaced. Such a child might refuse to stay in bed during bedtime or may exhibit some behavioral problems.

Before and after a new sibling arrives, make sure the child continues his usual bedtime routines. You should try as much as possible to take part in bedtime activities that require your presence. This will go a long way in preventing bedtime problems. Also, if the older sibling sleeps in the same room as you, it might be better not to move him out. You should try to make things stay the same for your older child. For toddlers especially, you can tell the child he can stay in the room as long as he doesn't disturb his baby sibling. You should make him excited about getting a new sibling.

If you need the crib for the new baby, and the older sibling is old enough to sleep in a bed, make sure the child is aware before moving him. You can make the transition before the new sibling arrives. It can also be accompanied with a reward system to motivate the child. After the new sibling arrives, you may need the help of other members of the household, as attending to multiple children alone isn't easy. Also, you can get a white noise machine to drown out household sounds to help your baby sleep better.

If some methods do not work, can you try them later?

There may be situations where it looks like a sleep training method isn't working. If that is the case, there are some things you should confirm first. The first is if the sleep training method is suitable for the baby. Sometimes, the method you adopted might not suit your baby's temperament. In that case, the method won't work no matter how long you apply it. The second thing to check is if there are any health or developmental issues affecting the child's sleep. Medical issues, some of which we have examined before, can affect the child's sleep patterns, thereby making it look as if a sleep training method is ineffective. If there are any health issues, then you need to treat that first.

Also, the issue might be inconsistency or failing to apply the method correctly. If you aren't consistent with a method, it might be inconvenient for the child thereby making the method ineffective. After checking all these, the results will then determine your next line of action. If the method isn't suitable for your child, then you should choose another. If there's a medical issue causing problems, then you need to treat it first, after which you can continue using the sleep training method provided that it is suitable for your baby. Sometimes, you might need to give the baby more time to adjust; you just need to be consistent with it. However, if the sleep training method still doesn't work, you can try another or try at a later time. In some cases, the baby may just not be ready. You can either take a break then try it later, or you can try another suitable method after a while. Remember, you shouldn't rush your child through many methods in a short period of time.

What happens to a baby long term if you don't pick her up right after she starts crying?

If you regularly wait for a short amount of time before attending to the baby once she starts crying, then your baby will learn to self-soothe quickly. This is the reason why the cry-it-out method is the fastest sleep training method. It helps the child learn how to self-soothe quicker than most other sleep training methods. Many experts have suggested that fussy crying may be a way for the baby to expend the excess energy so they can return to a calm state before sleeping. During this period, the baby may fuss for a short time for no clear reason. It's better to leave the baby for a while during these moments.

However, there is the need to strike a balance. Crying is a major way of communicating for babies and the longer you ignore your baby's cries, the less motivated he is to communicate with you. Also, studies have shown that babies shouldn't be left alone to cry for more than 20 minutes due to the risk of brain damage and some other health risks. Dr. Sears is one of the child experts in favor of the balanced approach. According to him, younger babies should be attended to quickly once their cries show there may be something wrong or if they need your attention. As the baby gets older, a slower response time is better to help him learn how to self-soothe.

Like we have said in previous sections, you need to study your baby to know what her cries mean. Is she hungry? Tired? Uncomfortable? Bored? Wet? Once you recognize what is wrong, you'll be able to generate a suitable response time. For newborn babies, you should attend to them as fast as possible.

What are the good ol' days tips for treating colic?

Colic is one of the problems that may affect sleep in children with no known cause and no specific treatment. There are only ways to manage the symptoms. However, there are some old home remedies for managing colic which most parents agree are useful. The first is to lay the baby on their tummy across your stomach or lap. This helps to soothe the baby and also helps him release gas. Another method is to hold the baby for long periods at the usual times he goes through the crying bouts. Keeping the baby in a repetitive motion has also been found to help. Baby swings can help do this. Immediately after feeding, hold the baby upright or carry him with his stomach close to your shoulder. This has been found to help prevent acid reflux and bloating.

Swaddling and white noise has also been recommended by many parents. The white noise helps to distract them while the swaddling helps to comfort the baby. Pacifiers or breastfeeding is also recommended by many mothers. Babies have a natural sucking reflex and often use sucking as a means to relieve themselves. Other home remedies include warm baths, massage, and a change of environment.

Does reading before bedtime help or not?

Reading is among the bedtime routines experts recommend. It offers lots of benefits to both the parent and the baby. Experts suggest reading often to a baby even if it looks like she doesn't understand. It greatly helps the child's language and speech development. **Reading before bedtime is a way to bond with your baby**, and once it has become a bedtime routine, it goes on for a long time. Reading before bedtime helps the baby's social and emotional development and it also helps to calm her down during bedtime. Reading to children also helps them develop communication skills faster as they pick up a lot during these bedtime stories.

Reading before bedtime has also been found to lower the child's stress levels, including the amount of the stress hormone cortisol in babies and toddlers. Experts have said this happens because of the close contact and soothing tone which is very comforting for the child. Reading before bed is one of the most recommended bedtime routines with lots of advantages.

Conclusion

We hope you've had a great ride and that you have found this book helpful. Now that you are armed with what you need to know about sleep training, we trust you will apply these methods and tips to help your baby get quality sleep. We urge you to maintain consistency and have lots of patience, as this is key to successful sleep training. With this, your child will be sleep trained in no time.

Best Wishes.

About The Author

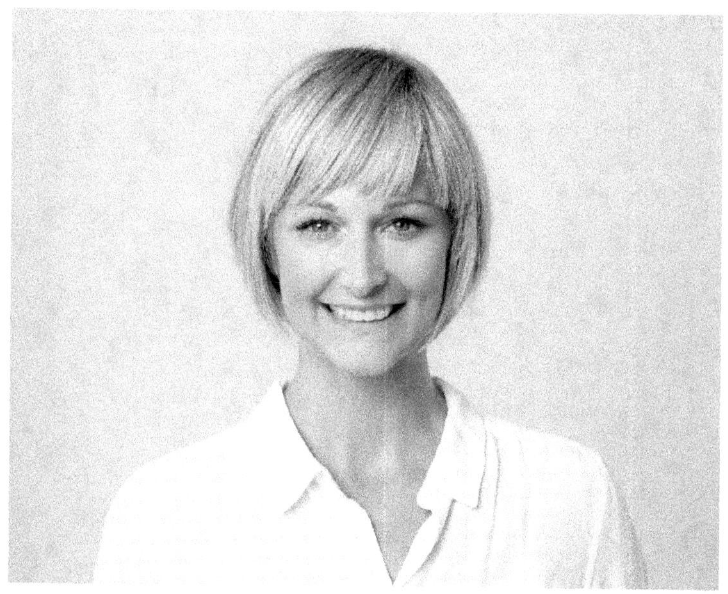

*M*ary Simmons graduated from Boston University in the faculty of social psychology and devoted herself to studying the problems of the relationship between children and adults, and has participated in research. As a member of several associations in Boston she aims at improving relations between children and has written articles on the upbringing of children in magazines and online publications. Mary has three children: 12, 5 and 2 years old. She sees her strongest achievement in sharing her own experience and skills to other people.

Please, leave a review !

I hope you enjoyed this book !

Reviews from awesome customers like you help others to feel confident about choosing this book too and navigate through their parenting times safely.

Please take a minute to share your experience !

I really appreciate it !

BONUS

Here's your bonus
http://marysimmonsbook.com/home/